GET SEXY, GIRLFRIEND!

Get Sexy, Girlfriend!

Your Ancestors Were Attractive, You Should Be Too

CANDI FRAZIER

HOUNDSTOOTH
PRESS

GET SEXY, GIRLFRIEND!
Your Ancestors Were Attractive, You Should Be Too

FIRST EDITION

ISBN   978-1-5445-5078-7 *Hardcover*
       978-1-5445-5077-0 *Paperback*
       978-1-5445-5079-4 *Ebook*

To the kids of future generations. I hope I'm not too late.

CONTENTS

DISCLAIMER

The information provided in this book is based on the personal experiences, opinions, and research of the author. It is not intended as medical advice, diagnosis, or treatment, and should not be construed as such. The author is not a licensed healthcare provider, and the content within this book is not a substitute for professional medical advice, treatment, or care. Always consult with a qualified healthcare provider before making any changes to your diet, exercise routine, or health practices, especially if you have underlying medical conditions or concerns. The author does not make any health claims, and the outcomes of following the information in this book may vary from person to person.

By reading this book, you agree that the author is not liable for any personal injury, health issues, or consequences that may arise from applying the information contained within.

STRONG LANGUAGE WARNING

Throughout this book, you'll notice that I don't shy away from strong language. My use of swear words is intentional—an expression of my authentic self and a refusal to adhere to outdated social norms that seek to suppress genuine communication. It's not about being edgy or shocking. It's about breaking free from the conditioning that tells us to censor ourselves. If some of the language offends you, I'm cool with that. I don't apologize for who I am, and I hope you'll embrace my honesty, unfiltered.

INTRODUCTION

Everything you think you know about health is a fucking lie.

And before you freak out—it's *not your fault, girlfriend.*

For decades, we were starved for information about how to take care of our bodies. We trusted doctors, food companies, and government agencies to tell us what was "healthy." And we believed them. We followed the food pyramid, jumped on the low-fat craze, counted calories like it was a religion, and thought whole grains were the holy grail of nutrition.

We did everything "right," and what did we get in return? A population that's fatter, sicker, more exhausted, and more disconnected from our wild, primal, sexy selves than ever before.

Now, we have the opposite problem: we're drowning in information.

Google any health question, and you'll get a thousand different answers, all contradicting each other. One expert says eat more protein, another says cut protein to extend your lifespan. One tells you carbs are killing you, another swears your thyroid will shut down without them. Veganism will save the planet! No, carnivorism will!

Oh, wait—have you tried carb cycling?

What about intermittent fasting?

Blue zones?

Macros?

Longevity hacks?

Biohacking?

It's *too fucking much*. We're drowning in health information, and instead of clarity, all it's created is confusion. Nobody knows what to believe anymore. The truth has become indiscernible, buried under layers of marketing, corporate interests, and a never-ending stream of conflicting bullshit.

None of that is an accident either.

If you're confused, you're easier to manipulate. If you don't know what's truly healthy, you'll keep buying whatever garbage they sell you, believing it's the answer. You'll keep popping the pills, drinking the shakes, and spinning your wheels in frustration while your health, vitality, and raw, untamed energy continue to nosedive.

But here's my little secret: you don't need a guru, a diet plan, or a supplement stack to reclaim your power. You just need to remember what your body already knows. Our ancestors were strong, radiant, and primal. In other words, they were sexy as hell. They lived in harmony with nature, and their bodies worked.

And that's what this book is all about.

THE FREE FALL: HOW WE GOT HERE

In Daniel Quinn's excellent novel *Ishmael*, he describes civilization as a skydiver plummeting toward the ground, mistaking the rush of air for flight. That's us right now when it comes to our health. We jumped out of the plane, expecting our parachute to open, but the parachute was broken.

We abandoned nature's principles a long time ago, convinced we could outsmart biology with lab-grown food, artificial light, and whatever the fuck the FDA is calling a "balanced diet" these days. We swapped real food for processed garbage, sunlight for blue light, movement for sedentary convenience, and deep, restorative sleep for Netflix binges.

And we're still smiling in free fall, wondering why we feel like shit.

Sluggishness, brain fog, bloating—these aren't "normal." They're symptoms of disconnection. Most people assume they're aging, not realizing they're comparing themselves to a sick, inflamed average. Then the crash happens: obesity, diabetes, autoimmune disorders, infertility.

Now they're scrambling for a parachute that doesn't exist.

At this point, people panic. They scramble for a fix—medications, miracle diets, or their favorite influencer's protocol. The solutions they reach for, however, are still inside the same broken system. A prescription can't reverse a lifetime of biological confusion. A detox tea won't undo years of missing sunlight, shitty sleep, and blood sugar chaos.

Just like in *Ishmael*, the damage is already done. There is no quick fix. You can't erase decades of disconnection overnight.

But, you can rebuild.

That's the good news, girlfriend: *your body is built to heal.* It is not beyond repair. It's been fighting for you this whole time—adapting, compensating, doing its best with what it's been given. And the moment you start giving it what it *actually* needs—real food, natural light, restorative sleep, movement, nature—it responds.

Our health wasn't always this complicated. Our ancestors didn't need nutrition labels or hormone panels to stay well. They didn't track macros or download apps to stay healthy. They just lived in alignment with nature, and their bodies worked.

So what changed?

Our world.

Our food.

But most critically, our *environment*.

And by environment, I don't mean pollution or what city you live in. Instead, it's everything your body is exposed to—your light environment, your food environment, your movement environment, your social environment, even your emotional environment. The air you breathe, the sounds you hear, the light hitting your skin, the temperature you sleep in, the way you wake up, the way you move, the way you eat—it's all part of your internal operating *environment*. And most of it is completely out of harmony with what your body was designed for.

This is why we're sick. We've become disconnected from the rhythms that once governed us. And now our bodies are screaming. Symptoms, diagnoses, and dysfunction—they're not random. They're messages. Your body is playing a constant game of hot-and-cold, trying to steer you back toward health. Unfortunately, most people just slap on a Band-Aid and keep moving, ignoring the cries for help.

Conditions like PCOS, insulin resistance, or thyroid issues are not random—they're red flags. Autoimmunity, cancer, and heart disease don't just happen either. They're the result of chronic misalignment with nature.

The most overlooked truth is that your body is nothing short of miraculous. It's resilient as hell—built to adapt, built to endure, built to survive even under *absolute shit conditions*. That's the only reason chronic symptoms show up in the first place. It's not your body failing—it's your body *fighting*, desperately trying to keep you alive despite living out of harmony with nature.

This book will show you how to stop fighting against your biology and start working with it. Not with fads or fear, but by remembering the principles that nature has for you.

NATURE BUILT YOU—AND SHE WANTS YOU BACK

You were born wild.

No algorithms, no macros, no tracking devices, just you and your raw human instinct. Your DNA is not synthetic. It was forged in relationship with the sun, the soil, the cold, the dark, and the food that once grew without labels.

And stepping outside that natural rhythm is killing us.

The moment you return, however—when you step barefoot onto the earth, soak in sunlight, breathe fresh air, eat real food, and move your body—something ancient wakes up. It's not just a mood boost, it's biology. When you feel that surge of energy, that hit of peace, that lift in your spirit, that's nature rewarding you for doing exactly what you were built to do.

We've tuned out that wisdom, though. We've traded that connection for screens, comfort, and convenience. We've ignored nature's signals and confused stillness with laziness, sickness with aging, and survival with health.

But you don't have to keep living that way. You don't need permission to reclaim your wild self. You just need to remember it.

This book isn't about reinventing your life. It's about remembering the one you were built for. When you strip away the noise and reconnect with the 7 Principles of Nature, your body remembers too. It knows how to heal, how to regenerate, and how to thrive.

In other words, it knows how to get sexy.

Sexiness isn't superficial. It's not about posing, pleasing, or fitting into someone else's mold. It's a *sign of health*. A sign that your hormones are balanced, your energy is high, and your skin is glowing. The outside starts to radiate what's happening on the inside. That's why getting sexy is something to strive for—not in spite of your age, but because of it.

And it's not only possible, it's inevitable when you live by nature's principles.

Because you were never meant to be tamed. You were made to look and feel fucking sexy!

WHAT YOU'LL LEARN

In this book—*Get Sexy, Girlfriend! Your Ancestors Were Attractive, You Should Be Too*—I'll show you how to do exactly that: return to the natural, vibrant, and yes, sexy state your body was built for. The version of yourself that nature intended. That version of you already exists. She's not buried under some genetic curse or locked away in some overpriced wellness retreat. She's just been hijacked by modern life, designed to keep you sick, sluggish, and dependent.

But you can take your power back. You don't need a miracle. You just need to follow the 7 Principles of Nature.

Now, these aren't my principles. I didn't invent them. *Nature did.* I simply learned to interpret them. These are the biological laws that have governed human health for millennia, long before food pyramids, calorie counting, and CrossFit. When you follow them, you wake up—mentally, physically, hormonally. You get your energy back. Your body starts working *for* you instead of *against* you. You get strong, sharp, and sexy as hell—not by dieting or biohacking yourself into oblivion, but by aligning with what your body craves.

I've dedicated each chapter to one of these principles:

- **Principle #1: Don't Fuck with Nature:** Nature has been running the show for millions of years. Your body is designed to work in sync with it. In this chapter, I expose the brutal truth: we've domesticated ourselves, just like we did to wolves, and every time we fuck with nature—whether in our food, environment, or daily habits—we pay the price in our genes, our health, and our vitality.

- **Principle #2: Don't Eat Clown Food:** If it didn't exist ten thousand years ago, it's not real food and your body wasn't built to digest it. Bananas and potatoes are sold as "healthy," but most modern food is glorified science fair garbage. In this chapter, you'll learn to eat like a human again, not a lab rat.

- **Principle #3: Find Joy Outside of Food:** Modern life has trained us to chase dopamine through snacks. If food is your main source of happiness, something's off. This chapter helps you build a life that actually feels good so you're not using cupcakes as a coping mechanism.

- **Principle #4: Master Your Body's Fuel System—or Stay Fat and Tired:** Your metabolism isn't broken; you just never learned how to use it. Your body was built to switch between burning glucose and fat. Once you unlock metabolic flexibility, you'll tap into steady energy, easier fat loss, and clearer thinking.

- **Principle #5: Worship the Sun:** You are, at least in part, solar-powered. Your mitochondria rely on sunlight to function and artificial light is scrambling your system. This chapter shows you how to reconnect with natural light and why the sun is more powerful than your multivitamin.
- **Principle #6: Obey Your Circadian Clock:** Your body has a built-in schedule, and when you eat, sleep, and move at the wrong times, your hormones rebel. Align with your circadian rhythm, and your body becomes a well-oiled machine. Ignore it, and you'll feel like you're running on fumes.
- **Principle #7: Reignite Your Sexy Hormones:** Your hormones are the power grid of your body—fueling your mood, metabolism, and sex drive. But modern stress, caffeine overload, and nutrient gaps are flipping the circuit breakers. This chapter helps you reconnect with your primal, pleasure-powered self.

These principles may seem like a lot, but as you'll see, they're not. They're simple, instinctive, and once you learn them, they'll stick. Not because they're revolutionary, but because they make sense. They feel true.

When you follow them, you'll stop fighting your body and start working with it. You'll have aha moments that change how you eat, sleep, move, and live—not out of discipline, but out of alignment.

You'll remember what it feels like to feed good, energized, clear, and alive. You'll stop surviving and start thriving.

Because when you live by nature, you get sexy.

HOW I RETURNED TO NATURE

Most of what I know about metabolic health, I learned from my husband, Tom.

Before we met, I was a board-certified functional nutritionist and medical professional nutrition educator and I'd spent over a decade helping thousands of women overcome health challenges. But the most common struggle—the one that came up again and again—was weight loss.

And I couldn't figure it out for myself either.

I did everything "right." Keto, carnivore, South Beach, HIIT, CrossFit, 75 Hard—you name it, I tried it. I trained hard. I was disciplined. And still, that stubborn layer of fat wouldn't budge.

I followed all the advice. I stuck to every plan. So why wasn't it working?

Then, I met Tom.

Tom is a type 1 diabetic. His pancreas doesn't produce insulin. I knew the textbook science of diabetes, insulin resistance, and blood sugar regulation, but watching someone live with it in real time was a whole different education.

His blood sugar dictated everything. I'll never forget the first time I saw him go low. His insulin pump—meant to act like a pancreas—overcorrected. And just like that, he crashed. Sweating, shaky, and crabby as hell. Panicking, I grabbed some maple syrup so he could get his blood sugar back up. It was not fun.

He told me he had learned to live with low blood sugar episodes—but looking back, he realized they happened far less often during periods he ate fewer carbohydrates. That's when we made a pact: to stabilize his blood sugar once and for all, with a highly focused, committed effort unlike anything he'd tried before.

So we got to work. We stripped away the variables. We ate low-carb. We tracked everything. We moved more, walked together, lifted weights. We built our days around keeping his blood sugar stable.

And it worked.

No spikes. No crashes. No drama. His blood sugar became a flat line of control and consistency. His A1C dropped to levels that barely registered as diabetic, all without more meds. Just nature—food, light, movement, and rhythm.

Every time we ate together, Tom needed insulin. And that's when it hit me—if *he* needed insulin for that food, so did I. The only difference? My pancreas was doing the work behind the scenes. Talk about a light bulb moment! I then started watching my own patterns—tracking meals, energy, workouts. I followed exactly what worked for him. Same meals, same movement. And within a month, I dropped thirteen pounds.

Thirteen pounds!

After years of struggling, that one shift shattered everything I thought I knew.

Tom just looked at me and said, "I told you, honey. The more *insulin* I take, the *fatter* I get. Insulin is a master fat-storing hormone." He had always known. "It's just that black- and-white."

I had been overcomplicating what was really very simple: the more your body needs insulin, the harder it is to burn fat. From that point on, I was obsessed. I tracked his food, his insulin, his glycogen stores, his ketones. I watched patterns emerge and saw the truth that no textbook or expert had ever taught me. Helping him manage his blood sugar gave me front-row insight into the metabolic blueprint every woman needs.

And that's how our wildly successful weight-loss business, Primal Bod, was born—its name rooted in the realization that what we'd discovered was perfectly aligned with how our ancestors lived.

Together, Tom and I turned everything we learned into a system—a primal, no-BS approach to effortless fat loss and lifelong health. We started sharing it with clients, and the results were jaw-dropping. Hundreds of women were waking up to a whole new way of living—one that made sense, felt good, and actually worked. As of the writing of this book, we've helped more than six thousand women (in less than eighteen months!).

This book is part of that mission.

Some people call me a social media influencer. And hey, I get it—I post about my life, share what works, and yes, I have an audience. But Tom and I did not get into this for the likes or the brand deals. Influencers chase attention, then figure out how to cash in on it.

That's not me. I'm just wildly obsessed with this lifestyle because it changed my life—and now I can't shut up about it. Tom and I, we like to think of ourselves more as enthusiasts with a platform.

We live primal-y because it works. And if it works for you too? Even better.

WHY I WROTE THIS BOOK

I wrote this book because the world has made health way too complicated. If you're tired of the confusion, the frustration, and the endless cycle of trying things that don't work, you're in the right place.

This isn't about hacks, trends, or diet fads. It's not a set of macros, a meal plan, or a rigid list of "good" and "bad" foods either. It's something far more powerful: a return to nature.

The way we've been taught to think about food, health, and our bodies is backward. This book is here to break the conditioning. To teach you how to reconnect to what you already know deep down: your body was never the problem. It's the modern world that's out of alignment.

And no, I won't be sharing the Primal Bod program within these pages; my wildly successful weight loss program doesn't translate well to a static book format. It's interactive by design. What I'm sharing here is bigger. This book is about nature: the rhythms, principles, and signals that have guided human health for millennia. And how to navigate a world that's pulled you away from it all.

Throughout these pages, you'll also occasionally hear directly from Tom. As a type 1 diabetic, his lived experience with blood sugar management shaped much of what we teach—and in some moments, it makes more sense for those insights to come straight from him.

You certainly don't need more information. Instead, you need clarity, truth, and simplicity. And you need to stop giving your power to experts who profit off your confusion.

When you understand the *why* behind your biology, you stop chasing the next big thing. You stop micromanaging every bite of food. You stop falling for the lie that your health is too complicated to figure out for yourself (yes, there are exceptions here). Instead, you start making aligned choices. You start trusting your body. You start living like a woman who was built to thrive. The goal isn't perfection. It's alignment. Because when you live in harmony with nature, your body works.

You don't need another diet. You need to remember that sexy isn't reserved for the young, the Photoshopped, or the genetically blessed. Sexy is health. Sexy is harmony. Sexy is feeling strong in your body, lit up in your life, and deeply connected to the truth of who you are.

I've seen women in their forties, fifties, and sixties feel sexier than they ever did in their twenties—not because of what they lost, but because of what they reclaimed. Their energy. Their confidence. Their wild, radiant selves.

And that's what this book is here to help you do.

Let's dive in.

DON'T FUCK WITH NATURE

Nature doesn't negotiate—and every time we fuck with it, we pay the price.

Back in the 1930s and '40s, Dr. Francis M. Pottenger Jr. ran a study that should've slapped some sense into how we think about food and its impact on generational health. His research wasn't just a wake-up call back then; it was a full-on siren warning us what happens when you mess with nature.

At the time, Pottenger was studying tuberculosis, particularly the role of adrenal glands in fighting the disease. To study this, Pottenger performed adrenalectomies—removing the adrenal glands—on cats. It was grueling, meticulous work.

As word got out that he was using cats for his research, people started donating their cats to the cause. Suddenly, Pottenger had more cats than he knew what to do with, and that led to a new problem: feeding them.

At first, it was manageable. He fed the cats what they were built to eat—a diet of raw meat, raw milk, and other unprocessed foods.

These cats thrived, even after the stress of surgery. They recovered quickly, had sleek coats, strong bones, and an overall vitality that couldn't be ignored.

But as the number of cats grew, his supply of raw food started to dwindle. He was forced to cut corners, substituting cooked meats, sweetened condensed milk, and other processed scraps for some of the cats. And that's when things started to unravel. The processed-fed cats became weak and sickly, struggling to recover from surgery. Pottenger couldn't help but notice the stark difference between the thriving raw-fed cats and their ailing, processed-fed counterparts.

What started as a logistical headache turned into a groundbreaking study. Pottenger was intrigued and—being the scientist that he was—decided to explore some more. He split the cats into groups and fed them six different diets ranging from completely raw to fully processed.

The results weren't just dramatic; they were devastating.

On one end of the spectrum, the cats on the raw diet stayed healthy and strong, generation after generation. Their bones were dense, their teeth aligned perfectly, and their coats practically glowed. But the ones eating only processed foods? By the second generation, they were falling apart. Skeletal deformities, fertility issues, and hormonal imbalances were rampant. By the third generation, these cats were plagued with disease, and by the fourth, they couldn't reproduce. Their immune systems collapsed, parasites moved in, and males and females started displaying opposite-sex traits (females turned aggressive; males became passive).

Why does this matter? Because the same thing is currently happening to us.

While Pottenger's cats were fed processed scraps and their health crumbled, we humans are doing far worse. While those cats deteriorated on cooked meat and condensed milk, we've taken it to another level entirely. It's not just what we're eating; *it's how we're living.*

We've removed ourselves so far from nature that the very things designed to keep us alive—clean air, natural light, nutrient-dense food—are now replaced by chemical-laden air fresheners, LED screens, and fortified junk. We've gone beyond messing with our diet; we've messed with every element of nature that supports life.

Like Pottenger's cats, we've built a world that works against our biology.

In other words, we've fucked with nature, and it's time to knock that shit off.

In this chapter, we'll explore what happens when we mess with nature's blueprint—how we didn't just domesticate plants and animals, but ourselves. By eliminating scarcity and engineering a cozy world of abundance, we've wrecked our metabolism, hormones, and instincts, making us softer, sicker, and more dependent than ever. You'll also learn about how our genes have been hijacked, why modern medicine keeps us alive but not thriving, and how the comforts we've created have turned into our cages.

DOMESTICATION: FROM WOLVES TO CHIHUAHUAS

When people think of domestication, they usually think of dogs. It's the most obvious example—the one sitting right in their house, wagging its tail, begging for scraps. Most people know that dogs were bred from their wild counterpart, the wolf.

A wolf is a perfect, efficient, wild predator—built for endurance, survival, and the hunt. Some dog breeds have retained their working instincts, bred to herd, guard, or retrieve. But others? Not so much. Take the chihuahua, for example. It's about as far from a wolf as you can get. It shakes when it's cold. It barks at shadows. If you threw it into the wild, it wouldn't last a fucking day. It would either freeze to death or become a snack for a hawk.

So, why is this descendant from a wolf such a weakling?

Because we bred the survival out of it.

We took a wild predator and selectively bred it for convenience, aesthetics, and submission. Wolves hunt, work in packs, and survive on their own. Chihuahuas sit in handbags. They've been tamed, softened, made dependent.

That's domestication.

And while it's easy to see domestication in dogs, we've done the exact same thing to our food. Virtually every plant we eat today has been engineered—not by nature, but by us. (I'll dive even deeper into how selective breeding has shaped food in the next chapter.)

And let's not overlook alcohol. Early civilizations figured out that fermented grains and fruit made booze—and that became a major driver of crop selection. Corn? Perfect for whiskey. Wheat? Great for beer. Fruits? Ideal for wine. The push to grow these crops wasn't about nutrition—it was about getting drunk.

We took wild plants, made them sweeter, softer, and easier to grow, and then called it an improvement. But in reality, we fucked with nature.

And now, we're paying the price.

DOMESTICATION VS. SELECTIVE BREEDING

Let's back up for a second, because in my experience, people get tripped up on the words "domestication" and "selective breeding." Up to this point, we've talked about how we domesticated dogs and selectively bred plants, but these two concepts aren't interchangeable. People assume domestication only applies to animals—especially dogs—but it's much bigger than that. Domestication isn't just about breeding; it's about fundamentally altering an organism's nature, making it more dependent, more controllable, and often less resilient in the wild.

Selective breeding, on the other hand, is about choosing specific traits over generations—whether for size, temperament, yield, or taste. And while domestication and selective breeding overlap, how we apply them to plants and animals is wildly different.

When we selectively breed plants, for example, we splice genes, alter DNA, and create crops that wouldn't survive in the wild. Many modern fruits and vegetables are sterile—they can't reproduce without human intervention. Those "wild" pineapples and mangoes in

Costa Rica are not wild at all. They've been genetically manipulated for sugar consumption. They may look natural, but they're domesticated food, just like store-bought tomatoes or seedless grapes.

Now compare that to animals, particularly livestock. Yes, we selectively breed farm animals, but we're not splicing their genes in a lab. Instead, we breed the strongest, healthiest animals together to produce better offspring.

Modern meat started as food—and it's stayed food. Modern plants, on the other hand, started as toxic fibers growing from the ground.

As a result, meat, for the most part, remains closer to its natural form. Most of the meat we eat hasn't been tampered with on the same level as fruits and vegetables. Yes, there are exceptions—like Impossible Burger, a lab-engineered "meat" designed to mimic the real thing but built entirely from processed plant oils, soy, and synthetic additives. But overall, real meat, specifically wild animals and organically raised livestock, remains relatively untouched compared to the lab-level manipulation happening with crops.

When it comes to plants, we've hacked their DNA beyond recognition.

The reason I am pointing this out is because our genes haven't had time to catch up with these new creations. It's taken us millions of years to adapt to the foods that were available in nature. Now, in the blink of an eye—just ten thousand years—we're throwing new foods into our bodies that we were never designed to process (more on this in a bit). The fruits, grains, and vegetables you're eating now are the result of man's tinkering, not nature's design. It's a science experiment conducted on a grand scale marketed with bright colors and fancy packaging.

WE ARE THE NEW DOMESTICATED SPECIES

Domestication didn't stop at plants and animals either. Every species we've domesticated has lost something in the process—strength, resilience, independence. And as we reshaped the world around us, we unknowingly did the same to ourselves.

We are the new domesticated species.

Look at a modern human compared to a hunter-gatherer from twenty thousand years ago:

- We are softer, weaker, fatter, and more dependent than ever.
- We're physically smaller. Farming made humans shorter, more fragile, and prone to disease.
- Our brains have shrunk. Yep, the human brain is smaller than it was ten thousand years ago.
- We've lost common sense. Our ancestors could track animals, navigate without a map, and survive in the wild. Most people today can't even start a fire.
- We are completely dependent. Our food comes from stores, our water from taps, and without these systems, most of us wouldn't last a week.

Just like we bred wolves into chihuahuas, we have bred ourselves into *Homo familiarus*—the domesticated human.

How did we fuck with nature to get here? Well, it started with the Agricultural Revolution.

The Agricultural Shift: The First Major Fuck-Up

For hundreds of thousands of years, humans lived as hunter-gatherers. We moved with the seasons, ate what was available, and adapted to our environment. Our diets were high in animal protein and fat, supplemented with whatever plants we could forage. We were metabolically flexible, lean, strong, and built for endurance.

Then we got "smart."

Roughly ten thousand years ago, we stopped roaming and started farming. The Agricultural Revolution was supposed to be humanity's great leap forward, but from a health perspective, it was the first domino in a chain of disastrous decisions. Instead of a diverse diet rich in nutrients, we became dependent on grains—calorie-dense, but nutritionally weak compared to the meat and fat we once thrived on (not to mention the impact on our blood sugar!).

And the consequences showed up fast.

Archaeological evidence paints a stark picture. Compared to their hunter-gatherer ancestors, early crop farmers were shorter, had weaker bones, and suffered from more dental issues. They had more infections, more nutrient deficiencies, and a lower overall quality of life. Their grain-heavy diet led to metabolic dysfunction, and their sedentary lifestyles made them physically weaker.

We see this pattern again and again in history. The moment a society shifts from hunting and gathering to farming crops, health declines.

Take the Mongols, for example. These nomadic warriors lived off of meat, dairy, and animal fat. They were bigger, faster, and stronger than their agricultural neighbors. When they swept through Asia and Europe, they dominated settled farming populations who were physically weaker and less resilient. The same goes for other warrior cultures—like the Maasai in Africa and the Inuit in the Arctic—who continue to thrive on animal-based diets and have historically outperformed agricultural societies in both strength and endurance.

So why did we stick with agriculture if it made us weaker?

Because it made food *predictable.*

Farming provided stability. Instead of relying on the hunt, people could grow food and store it. They could settle in one place, build villages, and raise families without worrying about starvation. It was a trade-off: we gave up health in exchange for security.

And over time, we adapted—to an extent. Our bodies learned to tolerate grains, but we never thrived on them. Compared to our hunter-gatherer ancestors, we are still smaller, sicker, and more prone to disease. The human body wasn't designed to process large amounts of carbohydrates every day, yet we built entire civilizations around them.

The Agricultural Revolution didn't just change what we ate—it changed who we were.

Just like wolves became dogs through selective breeding, humans changed in response to our new environment. We became less physically robust, more dependent on outside resources, and more susceptible to disease. The self-sufficiency of our hunter-gatherer past was replaced with reliance on farming, trade, and eventually, industry.

We laid the foundation for everything that would come next—the industrialization of food.

The Industrial Food Era: The Real Disaster Begins

If the Agricultural Revolution was humanity's first major health fuck up, the Industrial Revolution was the one that put the nail in the coffin. Farming may have weakened us, but at least our ancestors were still eating real food—just too much grain and not enough meat. But once we industrialized food production? That's when things really went off the rails.

This is when we stopped just tampering with nature and started full-on engineering it.

With factories came mass production. With mass production came efficiency. And with efficiency came profit-driven, chemically altered, artificially processed food-like substances that looked like food, smelled like food, and tasted like food but nutritionally were complete garbage.

Before the Industrial Revolution, food was grown, raised, or hunted. Sure, farming had its flaws, but at least wheat was wheat and milk was milk. But after we figured out how to refine, strip, bleach, fortify, and chemically alter food for a longer shelf life, everything changed. We stopped eating whole foods and started eating processed foods.

- Refined sugar and white flour became dietary staples.
- Cheap vegetable oils replaced animal fats.

- Artificial preservatives and additives were introduced to make food last longer and look more appealing.

For the first time in human history, we had calories without nutrients.

And instead of recognizing the problem, we doubled down. We started removing more and more of the natural elements in our food—stripping it of minerals and vitamins—and then fortifying it with synthetic versions because it was making people sick.

Think about that. We took food, stripped it of its nutrients, and then had to artificially add them back in to keep people alive. Talk about fucking with nature.

But wait, there's more!

It wasn't just food processing that fucked us over. We also industrialized the way we raised our food. Instead of raising animals the way nature intended, we packed them into feedlots, pumped them full of grains, antibiotics, and hormones, and turned what was once nutrient-dense, grass-fed meat into a sickly, hormone-laden product that barely resembled its wild counterpart.

- Cows stopped eating grass and started eating corn and soy, leading to meat that's inflamed and nutritionally inferior.
- Chickens were bred to grow twice as fast, making their meat higher in omega-6 inflammatory fats and lower in quality.
- Pigs were confined to pens, growing unnaturally fat and weak.

Sound familiar? We did the same thing to plants. We genetically modified them to grow bigger, faster, and cheaper—which meant less nutrition per bite and more exposure to pesticides and chemicals.

Today, we're eating more food than ever, but getting less nutrition than ever. When I see an obese person these days, I don't just see their excess weight. I see profound degrees of protein deficiency and signs of the disease: bulbous noses, reddened skin, swollen (edematous) ankles, and countless other subtle but telling cues that the body is deeply unwell.

At this point in our history, food wasn't just food anymore: it was *a business*. The goal wasn't to nourish people; it was to sell as much as possible. So they did exactly what any smart business does: they made their product addictive. They manipulated flavors to make processed foods hyperpalatable. They added sugar, salt, and fat in perfect ratios to keep your brain coming back for more.

And then they marketed the hell out of it.

They slapped words like "heart-healthy," "low-fat," "natural," and "organic" on boxes to make people think they were making smart choices. They got government agencies and health organizations to back them up. They infiltrated schools, hospitals, and food guidelines.

And now people don't even know what real food is anymore. We're fatter, sicker, and more exhausted than ever. And instead of fixing the problem, they just sell us more solutions—pills, supplements, diet plans, and medical treatments.

If all of that isn't fucking with nature, I don't know what is.

THE DEATH OF SCARCITY: HOW WE BECAME DOMESTICATED

For hundreds of thousands of years—before the agricultural and industrial revolutions—scarcity was the rule. It dictated everything: when we ate, what we ate, and how much effort it took to get food in the first place.

Meat was the ultimate prize, the most nutrient-dense fuel our bodies could get. But it wasn't easy. Hunting required skill, strategy, and sometimes days of tracking before a successful kill. Because of that, our ancestors didn't take it for granted—they built their entire existence around securing it. When the hunt failed, our ancestors turned to plants, not because they were optimal, but because they were better than starving. And even then, wild plants weren't the sugar-loaded, oversized versions we see today. They were tough, fibrous, and often bitter, with just enough calories to keep someone alive until real food (meat) became available again.

Scarcity kept everything in balance. It ensured that food was something earned—not something endlessly available—and it shaped human metabolism to thrive in cycles of feasting and famine.

It wasn't just about food either. Scarcity was a biological guardrail that shaped human evolution. It ensured we didn't overconsume. Physical effort kept us strong and resilient. Seasonal rhythms dictated what we could gather, hunt, or harvest at any given time. These weren't limitations; they were nature's way of keeping us in harmony with the world around us.

These guardrails were a gift.

They didn't just determine what we ate; they shaped who we became. Our metabolism, our hormones, our instincts—they were all honed under these constraints, forcing us to adapt, endure, and thrive in a world where food wasn't guaranteed.

Scarcity built us.

But again, this is when we got "smart." Human ingenuity stepped in, and scarcity disappeared overnight.

Agriculture gave us an abundance of grains. Processing made foods last longer, taste sweeter, and require less effort. Modern transportation brought out-of-season fruits to our tables year-round. Industrialization brought us refined sugars and ultraprocessed foods by the truckload. Suddenly, we weren't foraging or hunting—we were stockpiling. We weren't fasting between kills—we were grazing all day. We weren't working for our food—we were ordering it from the couch. The world we adapted for—the one that shaped our metabolism, our instincts, and our very biology—was gone.

And with it, the natural constraints that kept us in check. Scarcity? Eliminated by endless grocery store aisles and 24/7 drive-throughs. Physical effort? Replaced by machines, delivery apps, and sedentary lifestyles. Seasonal eating? A distant memory when you can buy strawberries in December and pineapple whenever the fuck you feel like it.

At first glance, this seems like a win. No more famine. No more feast-or-famine cycles. No more struggling to find food. But scarcity wasn't just an inconvenience—it was a *governing force of nature*.

Remove scarcity from the equation, and everything breaks down. Our bodies weren't designed for endless food on demand. We weren't meant to eat year-round like winter never comes. We weren't meant to have sugar and carbohydrates available every time we opened the pantry. But now we do.

We have become domesticated.

We've eliminated every natural barrier that once kept us in balance, and now we're paying for it. And it happened because we manipulated nature instead of working with it.

HOW WE'VE FUCKED WITH OUR GENES

When we abandoned nature's guardrails, we didn't just screw ourselves over, we set off a chain reaction that's still unfolding. Because what we eat doesn't just affect us; it affects the generations that come after us.

What you put in your mouth today isn't just shaping your *body*; it's shaping your *bloodline*. It's either strengthening it or setting it up for failure. Food isn't just fuel—it's information. Every bite sends signals to your DNA, flipping epigenetic switches that control immune function, fertility, metabolism, and longevity.

These switches don't reset when you're done eating; they carry forward, amplifying the damage with each generation. This is why we're seeing skyrocketing rates of chronic illness, infertility, and developmental disorders—not just in adults, but in kids born into a world saturated with modern-day toxicity, stripped of the natural conditions that once kept us resilient.

And even though the human body is built to adapt, it needs time to do so.

For millions of years, our genes evolved in response to slow, natural changes. When early humans first migrated out of Africa into northern regions with weaker sunlight, their skin gradually lightened over generations to absorb more vitamin D. This adaptation helped prevent deficiencies in environments where sunlight was scarce. Similarly, as these populations encountered seasonal variations in food availability, their metabolisms adjusted to store and use energy efficiently. Our bodies were constantly fine-tuning themselves to match the environment, keeping us lean, strong, and adaptable.

But in the last few centuries—hell, even since the 1950s—things changed. We went from an ancestral diet of meat and animal fat to a diet of sugar-filled garbage. We went from natural rhythms dictated by the sun to artificial light blasting us 24/7. We traded seasons of scarcity for unlimited food, climate-controlled comfort, and a life that requires zero physical effort.

That's a genetic shock our bodies weren't built for.

Adaptation takes time—thousands of years. But we've flipped the script overnight, and now we're dealing with the fallout.

EPIGENETICS: WHY YOUR GENES AREN'T YOUR DESTINY

For years, people have been spoon-fed the idea that their health is written in their DNA: "If your parents had heart disease, cancer, or diabetes, then you're doomed to get it too." That outdated view has been great for fear-based marketing and corporate profits, but it's dead fucking wrong.

Our genes are not the problem. The problem is how we're triggering them.

Welcome to epigenetics—the science that turns that whole narrative on its head. Yes, you inherit your genes from your parents. That part is nonnegotiable. But whether those genes actually *express* themselves—whether they make you sick or keep you strong—is largely up to you.

Your daily choices—the food you eat, the stress you carry, the light you expose yourself to, the way you move (or don't move)—are flipping epigenetic switches on or off all the time. Even the American Cancer Society acknowledges that only 5 to 10 percent of cancers are purely genetic. That means up to 95 percent of cancers are not dictated by your genes—it is a choice. I know that sounds bold—no one would *choose* cancer—but that's exactly the point. Most people don't realize they're making those choices until it's too late.

Yet, people still love to say, "Well, cancer runs in my family."

Does it, though? Or does eating a ton of sugar (or carbohydrates) run in your family? Does sitting on the couch every night run in your family? Does never seeing the sun and being constantly inflamed run in your family?

We're not passing down a genetic curse; we're passing down laziness. Families don't just share DNA, they share habits. The smoking habits, the processed food choices, the ice cream before bed—it all adds up over generations.

Your genes are only part of the equation. The real question is: *What are you doing to make sure they're working for you, not against you?*

(Note: Tom and I know some readers may have experienced cancer themselves. You have our deepest empathy and our sincere wishes for continued healing. If you're reading this book, it means you haven't given your power away—and we honor that. And yes, we fully acknowledge that in 5 to 10 percent of cases, cancer has nothing to do with personal choices.)

GENETIC VICTIMIZATION: THE ULTIMATE COP-OUT

The lie that "Your health is written in your DNA" isn't just false—it's dangerous. But honestly, for most people, it's also convenient.

If you believe your health is entirely dictated by your genes, then you don't have to change a damn thing. You can keep eating ice cream every night. You can pound margaritas on the weekends. You can scarf down oxalate-loaded foods while blaming your kidney stones on genetics. It's easier to believe that fate dealt you a bad hand than to confront the reality that your choices play a bigger role than you'd like to admit.

People would rather play the victim than the protagonist—an interesting outcome of a decadent society.

I call it "genetic victimization"—a bullshit excuse people cling to so they can avoid taking responsibility for their choices. Instead of questioning their diet, lifestyle, or habits, they chalk up their health issues to bad luck. It's easier to say chronic disease runs in the family than to acknowledge decades of poor eating and inactivity. Even cancer—while complex—is overwhelmingly influenced by environmental and lifestyle factors, with only a small fraction being purely genetic.

I get it, though. The human brain is wired for efficiency. It seeks the path of least resistance, conserving energy wherever possible. That's why people gravitate toward simple, one-variable answers. They require less thinking, less effort, and no real change.

And "It's just my genes" is the ultimate lazy answer.

It means you don't have to think deeper. It gives people permission to keep doing what they've always done, to stay comfortable, to avoid the hard work of reevaluating their choices. But life doesn't work like that, and your health sure as hell doesn't either. There's no single factor controlling your fate—your body is the result of every decision you make, every bite you take, every habit you build or break. Blaming genetics might feel easier in the short term, but in the long run, it's robbing you of control over your own life.

OTHER SIGNS WE'VE FUCKED WITH NATURE

It's one thing to acknowledge that we've strayed from nature's blueprint. It's another to realize just how much we've had to compensate for it.

Take biohacking, for example. The fact that biohacking even exists is a flashing red sign that we've fucked with nature. We've gotten so far removed from the way humans are supposed to live that we now have to engineer artificial solutions just to feel normal.

We wear blue light glasses because we bombard ourselves with artificial light from sunrise to sunset. We take ice baths because we never experience the cold. We choke down lab-formulated supplements because our food is nutritionally bankrupt.

And listen—I'm not saying you shouldn't do these things. In today's world, they're often necessary. Blocking blue light at night supports your circadian rhythm. Cold exposure boosts resilience and metabolic health. Fasting stimulates scarcity and helps reset your biology. Tom and I do these things too. The problem isn't that we are doing them—the problem is that we *have* to.

Biohacking isn't innovation, it's compensation. It's what happens when we disrupt nature so badly that we have to manufacture fake scarcity, fake cold exposure, fake nutrients—just to trick our bodies into working the way they were originally designed to.

This is just one of many signs we've fucked with nature.

We don't have real scarcity anymore, so we simulate it. We don't have real connection to nature, so we hack our way to a synthetic version of it. And all the while, we convince ourselves that this is just how things are. But take a step back, and it's clear: this world we've built—the one that's so abundant, so convenient, so comfortable—is completely unnatural.

And the consequences don't just stop with us.

MODERN DOGS, MODERN DISEASES: A REFLECTION OF OURSELVES

We aren't the only species paying the price for modern living. Every animal we've domesticated has suffered the same fate—our pets included. I'm circling back to dogs because, out of all the animals we've domesticated, they mirror us the most—and not just in companionship, but in the diseases we share.

Modern domesticated dogs are riddled with chronic diseases— arthritis, kidney disease, obesity, diabetes, inflammatory bowel disease, Addison's disease, allergies, epilepsy, cancer, heart disease, glaucoma, hypothyroidism, eczema. Sound familiar? These are the same ailments plaguing humans today.

Now, look at wolves. What do they die from? Parvo, rabies, Lyme disease, lice, distemper—acute infections, immune challenges, bacterial or viral threats. Not cancer. Not heart disease. Not diabetes. A wolf's death is dictated by nature, not by a slow, chronic deterioration caused by a mismatched diet and lifestyle.

This isn't a coincidence. We're feeding our dogs processed kibble—

loaded with grains and plant-based fillers their biology was never designed to handle—and now they're suffering from the same degenerative diseases we are.

It's Pottenger's cats all over again.

When animals (including us) are fed the wrong diet, generation after generation, their health collapses. Their bones weaken. Their fertility declines. Chronic disease sets in.

Wake up, girlfriend: We're doing the same thing to ourselves. We've domesticated ourselves, moved away from our natural diet, and replaced it with food-like substances that our bodies were never built to process. We're living longer but getting sicker, trapped in a slow-motion decline that looks a lot like the domesticated dogs limping to the vet.

This leaves us with a choice: we can die from nature's challenges—acute and natural—or we can suffer the slow, miserable decline of chronic disease brought on by ignoring what our bodies are designed for.

Daniel Vitalis makes the argument perfectly: the longest-living tiger on record was a twenty-six-year-old in a zoo, while wild tigers typically live around nine years. His response? "I'd rather live nine years in the wild than twenty-six in the zoo."

I couldn't agree more.

The same could be said for us. Living longer in a compromised state isn't the same as living well—which brings me to the next lie we've been sold: the idea that modern humans are healthier just because we're living longer.

LIFESPAN VS. HEALTHSPAN: LIVING LONGER, BUT NOT BETTER

One of the biggest arguments people make when defending modern life is "But we're living longer now!" Sure, the average life expectancy has increased, but that doesn't mean we're thriving. It doesn't mean we're living as nature intended. And the statistics are misleading.

A huge part of why life expectancy has risen isn't because we've mastered health—it's because we've reduced infant mortality. Historically, many children didn't survive childbirth and countless mothers died from complications. Modern medicine changed that with C-sections, neonatal care, and antibiotics. We also have emergency medicine for things that used to be death sentences—a broken leg in the wild, for example, meant you were done. Today, it's a minor inconvenience with a quick trip to the ER.

But while we've conquered traumatic and infectious causes of death, we've traded them for something worse: a slow, miserable decline into chronic disease. We're no longer dropping dead from infections or famines. Instead, we're being taken down by heart disease, cancer, diabetes, and autoimmune disorders—illnesses that barely existed when humans lived in sync with nature.

Ancient humans weren't dying early because they ate meat or lived a primal life. They were dying from accidents, poor sanitation, and childbirth complications. And let's not forget that a huge chunk of early deaths came at the hands of other humans—whether in a war, a duel, or a public execution.

Famine was another brutal force shaping human survival. When food was scarce, the weak didn't make it. Only the strongest genes were passed down. Today, however, we've removed scarcity, eliminated natural selection, and allowed everyone to survive and reproduce, resulting in a gene pool that's getting weaker, not stronger. Infertility is skyrocketing, chronic disease is everywhere, and immune systems are crumbling under the weight of modern living.

We've eliminated the sudden, dramatic deaths of the past, but at what cost? Yes, we're living longer—but not stronger, not healthier, and certainly not better. We've swapped "survival of the fittest" for "survival of everyone."

And the signs that we've fucked with nature are written all over our declining health.

WE'VE CREATED ZOOS FOR OURSELVES—
BUT WE CAN STILL BREAK OUT

In our relentless quest to make life easier, longer, and more comfortable, we've shaped not just our environment but ourselves. We started with animals—selectively breeding them for traits that suited our needs—but we didn't stop there. We engineered every aspect of life to remove hardship, discomfort, and struggle. We built a world where food is always available, shelter is climate-controlled, and medicine keeps us alive no matter how badly we treat ourselves.

And in doing so, we've built a cage.

Western medicine ensures we live longer. Sewage systems mean we don't have to worry about drinking water tainted with our own shit. Technology solved problems that once wiped us out. But when we removed nature's challenges, we also stripped away the very things that made us strong, adaptable, and connected to the world around us.

Now, we exist in a sanitized, over-engineered version of life. We shuffle from one comfort to the next, never hunting, never foraging, never struggling for anything beyond a Wi-Fi signal. We don't have to move, problem-solve, or even leave our homes. Tap a screen, and food appears at the door. Sit, eat, scroll, repeat. We call it normal.

But normal isn't natural.

This is what domestication has done to us. We've softened, become dependent, lost the instincts and resilience that once defined us. We are not wolves anymore. We are chihuahuas—fragile, anxious, and so far removed from our origins that we can barely function without a safety net. And the scariest part is that most people don't even realize it.

But here's the thing: awareness changes everything.

Once you see the cage, you can't unsee it. You start to notice how deep the domestication runs—how we've been shaped by a system that thrives on our dependence. Walk into a grocery store and really look. Look at the carts overflowing with ultraprocessed garbage. Look at the aisles stacked with products engineered for convenience, not nourishment. Look at the people debating which medication they need to manage the symptoms of a lifestyle disease they don't even realize they created.

Our ancestors didn't need pharmaceuticals. No one had a Prilosec deficiency.

The truth is, we no longer live in a world that forces us to overcome natural adversities. There was a time when, by fifteen or sixteen, you had real responsibilities within your tribe. You contributed, problem-solved, and faced challenges that built character and resilience. Now? We've eliminated every biological guardrail, removed every natural hardship, and created a world where people never have to struggle.

So how do you fix that? How do you escape a zoo you were born into?

You can't rewild yourself overnight, and you don't need to run off into the mountains and live off raw elk liver to break free. But you can start resisting domestication in small, meaningful ways. You can choose food that fuels you instead of weakens you. You can seek out discomfort instead of avoiding it. You can make the conscious decision to stop living like a caged animal—because here's the real difference between humans and every other domesticated species: we have a choice.

It won't be easy. The system is designed to keep you comfortable, compliant, and just numb enough not to question it. It takes discipline, effort, and a willingness to go against the grain. But when you do, you get something modern life has stripped away: strength, vitality, and the ability to thrive—not just exist.

Because the difference between being alive and truly living?

That's up to you.

DON'T EAT CLOWN FOOD

By now you know humans have been fucking with nature for a long time. We've bred wild plants into sugar bombs, manipulated animals for mass production, and engineered foods so far from their original form that they barely resemble what nature intended.

And yet, most people still think of "food" as whatever's sold at the grocery store—whether it's a bag of Cheetos or an organic apple. But just because it's edible doesn't mean it's real food.

When you hear "clown food," your mind probably jumps straight to the obvious offenders—McDonald's, Flaming Hot Cheetos, soy milk, and gas station nacho cheese. And yeah, those are absolute clown foods—no debate there. And I know you don't eat that shit. You're health-conscious. You shop organic. You avoid the drive-through. Maybe you've even sworn off alcohol.

That's great and all, girlfriend—but that's not what nature meant with this principle.

When I say "clown food," I'm not just calling out the obvious offenders like junk food or processed snacks. I don't need to waste your time with that; you already know this.

What I mean when I say "clown food" is *anything* that's been twisted, manipulated, or bred so far from its original form that it barely resembles what nature intended. Most of what's in your fridge, your pantry, and even your farmer's market stall is clown food.

That kale smoothie? Clown food.

Those vibrant heirloom tomatoes? Also clown food.

And don't get us started on fucking potatoes.

In this chapter, I'm breaking down what's real food and what's just a science experiment in disguise. While I'll expose plenty of clown food (though not all of it), this isn't just about what to avoid. It's about what to eat and why. I'll also dismantle the omnivore myth, prove why humans are built for meat, and explain how cows grow to be so fat. I'll then show you how to escape the modern food trap— what to eat, how to source real nutrients, and why fermented foods are more essential than ever.

But first, let's talk about clown food. If it didn't exist ten thousand years ago, it's not food—it's somebody's fucking science experiment.

Which begs the question: Are you a lab rat?

THE WORLD'S BIGGEST SCIENCE EXPERIMENT

If history has taught us anything, it's that every time humans mess with nature, we create unintended consequences. At first, it seems harmless—tweaking a plant to be a little sweeter, a little less bitter, a little more palatable. But fast-forward a few generations, and suddenly, we've got strawberries that can't survive without pesticides, bananas that can't reproduce, and tomatoes so fragile that nature itself seems determined to wipe them out.

This didn't happen overnight. Since 8000 BC, humans have been selectively breeding plants, cross-pollinating species, and forcing genetic changes to suit our needs. We saw this in the last chapter— how wild teosinte became modern corn, how tiny, fibrous apples turned into sugar-laden snacks, and how even "natural" produce is a human invention. That was just the warm-up. Now, we're diving deeper.

What started as a way to make plants edible quickly spiraled into something else. At first, it was about survival—taming wild plants so they wouldn't kill us. But once we gained control, we didn't stop at safety. We stripped away plant defenses, ramped up sugar content, and made food hyperpalatable. The further we got from the natural starting point, the more fucked-up things became.

The same selective breeding that once made wild foods edible has turned them into nutrient-poor, sugar-loaded, genetically fragile crops that can't survive without human intervention. Everything you see in the grocery store—or even the farmer's market—is a product of selective breeding. Bright orange carrots, crunchy cucumbers, smooth-skinned potatoes—none of them exist in nature. They've been engineered to be sweeter, less toxic, and more edible.

But even though we've tamed their flavors, they still carry plant toxins—their built-in chemical defenses against predators (including us).

Selective breeding sounds harmless, even natural, like we're just giving nature a helpful nudge. But when you radically alter a species' environment, you don't "improve" it—you create something that barely resembles its original form. It might still look like a plant, but its genetics have been so intensely manipulated that it's inching dangerously close to GMO territory.

People might argue, "Well, it's still a plant," but at what point does a plant stop being natural? It's time to crack open these preconceived notions.

CLOWN FOOD SCIENCE EXPERIMENTS

Let's start with almonds. Wild almonds were basically poison—fifty of them could kill a grown man. But ancient humans, being the experimental weirdos they were, figured out that if they stressed the almond tree just right—by cutting it open and shoving pine bark inside (who the fuck came up with that idea?)—it would stop producing such high levels of cyanide. Over time, through repeated manipulation, they turned a deadly nut into something edible.

And it wasn't just almonds. Humans have been forcing plants to conform to their preferences for thousands of years. Look at strawberries. Wild strawberries are tiny—about the size of a thimble—but they pack a punch in flavor. They were nature's perfect little gems. But then humans got greedy. They started selectively breeding them for size and sweetness, and today's modern strawberries are basically mutant sugar bombs. Even worse, they're so genetically altered that they can't survive in the wild. Farmers have to drench them in pesticides, fungicides, and herbicides just to keep them alive. Without these chemicals, modern strawberries wouldn't make it.

Cucumbers are another perfect example of how humans have been meddling with nature's design. Originally domesticated about eleven thousand years ago in Asia, the New World, and Africa, wild cucumbers were bitter and barely edible. Nobody with functioning taste buds wanted to eat them.

Even now, you can find wild cucumbers in Africa, where some of the world's last indigenous tribes still interact with them. In an episode of *The Outdoor Boys* on YouTube, Luke (the father) took his young kids to Africa to spend time with one of these tribes. The tribe would occasionally test wild cucumbers by licking or nibbling on them. Most of the time, they'd spit them out because they were too bitter to stomach. But if they stumbled upon a rare sweet one, they treated it like a small jackpot. But come the fuck on. Cucumbers were never a superfood. They were a survival food—something to eat when the hunt didn't go well. Modern cucumbers are completely different from their wild ancestors, so let's not pretend nature handed them to us in this form.

Then there are tomatoes. Originally, tomatoes were so toxic that people called them "stinking apples" or "poison apples." They belong to the nightshade family—known for its hallucinogenic and toxic properties—and early tomatoes were loaded with solanine, a natural toxin. Even today, green tomatoes and green potatoes can be dangerous if consumed in large amounts (more on potatoes coming up).

Some African tribes still eat a nightshade plant similar to tomatoes, but it's a risky move. Occasionally, people get seriously ill from eating them. The fact that humans even decided to eat tomatoes in the first place feels like a gamble that should've gone horribly wrong. But, of course, we intervened. Through selective breeding, humans engineered tomatoes to contain less solanine and more sugar, turning them into the sweet, juicy fruit we pile onto a plate of pasta.

And then there's the banana—the most genetically helpless fruit on the planet. The Cavendish banana, the one you see in every grocery store, can't reproduce on its own. They are sterile and seedless. Every Cavendish banana is a genetic clone of another, which makes its entire population susceptible to disease. Why? Because it's weak as fuck. Modern bananas are completely dependent on humans to exist. In contrast, wild bananas are rich in genetic diversity. They are tough, loaded with seeds, and capable of surviving in the wild because they've developed natural defenses over millennia.

Do you see a pattern here? Nature has rules. Plants are supposed to be resilient. Sugar is meant to be scarce. But we've overridden those natural balances and now modern fruits and vegetables are so weak that they require human intervention just to exist.

THE COST OF SUGAR: HOW IT RESHAPED OUR FOOD AND OUR BODIES

If there's one thing that has driven the manipulation of food more than anything else, it's sugar. The relentless push for more of it—whether for human consumption, alcohol production, or livestock feed—has reshaped agriculture, biology, and even civilization itself.

For thousands of years, humans lived in harmony with nature's natural checks and balances. Food was hard to come by, sugar was rare, and survival of the fittest ensured that only the strongest traits endured.

Whether you believe humans have been here for five thousand years or millions, one thing is true: our DNA adapted to *wild* food. Your body knew exactly what to do with a strawberry from twenty thousand years ago—tiny, tart, low in sugar, and barely enough calories to register. But today's strawberries? As you now know, they've been selectively bred into giant, sugar-loaded bombs that require pesticides and fumigants just to survive. They're no longer food—they're products.

This isn't just about strawberries. This is about *everything* we eat. Nature's slow, deliberate process of survival of the fittest was overridden in favor of mass production and profit. And sugar was the catalyst.

At first, sugar crops were manipulated to create alcohol. More sugar meant better, stronger fermentation, and as civilizations expanded—Egypt, Rome, and beyond—so did the demand for starchy, high-yield crops. Corn, wheat, barley, and potatoes were cultivated not because they were the most nutritious, but because they were *efficient*. They grew fast, they packed on weight, and they could feed an army or a workforce with minimal effort.

But it didn't stop with feeding *people*. Sugar-laden, starchy crops were also used to feed livestock—especially in the alcohol industry. The spent grains leftover from making beer and whiskey weren't tossed aside; they were fed to cows—cows that were never meant to eat grains in the first place.

Cows evolved to eat grass, not corn or barley. But grain-fattened cows put on weight quickly, which meant faster meat production. Unfortunately, their gut bacteria couldn't handle the diet. They developed infections, which spread to their milk, making people sick. Instead of stepping back and realizing *Hey, maybe feeding cows the byproducts of alcohol isn't a great idea*, the solution was to *pasteurize* the milk—boiling it to kill bacteria.

One unnatural intervention led to another, creating a food system so far removed from nature that the consequences—chronic disease, obesity, and metabolic dysfunction—became inevitable.

And that's the real cost of sugar. It wasn't just about satisfying a sweet tooth. It was about *controlling* food, *scaling* food, and *engineer-*

ing food for efficiency instead of health. It transformed agriculture, it shaped economies, and it created a system that no longer resembles the natural world our bodies were built for.

Every time we manipulated crops for sugar content—whether it was corn, wheat, or fruit—we took one more step away from nature's original design.

And the further we got, the sicker we became.

THE POTATO STORY: A LESSON IN PROGRAMMING, NOT JUST CROP MANIPULATION

The story of the potato isn't just about selective breeding; it's about how easily humans can be programmed to accept something as "food" when it suits those in power.

The potato, native to the Andean regions of South America, was introduced to Europe by Spanish explorers in the mid-sixteenth century. But when the Spaniards saw this strange tuber, their reaction was basically, *Hell no, we're not eating that.* The potato was widely distrusted and largely ignored, treated as an untrustworthy foreign object. It was only when starvation and control came into play that the narrative shifted.

In the eighteenth century, King Frederick II of Prussia, known as Frederick the Great, recognized the potato's potential to combat food shortages. His people were starving, and potatoes were cheap, easy to grow, and high-yielding. He first tested them on prisoners of war and hogs, watching as they managed to survive eating the starchy tubers. He then pushed potatoes as a staple food for his troops and country.

But the people weren't having it. In neighboring France, potatoes were outright illegal at the time because people believed eating them caused leprosy. And honestly, they were onto something. As previously mentioned, potatoes belong to the nightshade family, which contains solanine, a toxin that, in high enough doses (especially in green potatoes), can cause nausea, fever, skin lesions, muscle weakness, and even cardiac issues.

In other words, symptoms that look eerily similar to leprosy.

Frederick the Great's troops refused to eat them, famously saying, *The dogs won't even touch this shit!* But the king knew something about human psychology: if you tell people they *must* do something, they resist. But if you make them think *they're* the ones outsmarting the system, they'll jump at the opportunity.

So, he got clever. He built a walled compound where he planted potatoes and stationed armed guards around it, making it appear as though they were guarding something valuable. He then instructed his guards to occasionally (wink, wink) "fall asleep," allowing peasants to sneak in and steal the potatoes. Suddenly, potatoes weren't just food: they were *forbidden food*. And just like that, the peasants took the bait. They stole the potatoes, planted them, and before long, they were eating them willingly.

Antoine-Augustin Parmentier, one of Frederick's prisoners of war at the time, took this manipulation to the next level. As a pharmacist, he had survived on potatoes during captivity and realized they were an efficient, calorie-dense crop. Upon his release in 1763, he returned to France, which was facing a famine, and became the potato's biggest hype man. He lobbied tirelessly to get potatoes legalized, and in 1772, the French government lifted the ban.

But he didn't stop there. Parmentier needed the people to *want* potatoes, so he pulled a page straight out of Frederick's playbook. He hosted "potato parties," inviting high-profile guests—like Benjamin Franklin—to enjoy elaborate potato dishes. He gifted King Louis XVI and Marie Antoinette bouquets of potato blossoms to make them trendy. He even planted potatoes behind royal gates and staged "thefts" to make peasants *think* they were getting away with something exclusive.

And it worked. The very food that people once rejected out of fear became a staple crop—one that entire populations came to depend on.

So what's the point of this story?

It's not just about potatoes. It's about *you*.

Frederick's peasants were tricked into believing potatoes were valuable. They were conditioned into accepting a food they instinctively distrusted. They became *easy to control*. And if you think this kind of manipulation is a relic of the past, think again. It's happening *right now*.

Think about how many foods you've been told are "healthy" without ever questioning it. Whole grains. Oatmeal. Spinach. "Heart-healthy" vegetable oils. They stamp a label on a box and suddenly you assume it's good for you. But *who* is telling you it's good for you? Food corporations? Government agencies? The same people profiting off your confusion?

Our ancestors didn't need marketing campaigns to tell them what to eat. They didn't need a government-approved food pyramid or a stamp of approval from some corporate-backed nutritionist. They knew food wasn't food unless it was *real*, and even then, plants weren't the first choice; they were a last resort.

Plants like potatoes, tomatoes, and eggplants are all part of the nightshade family, which *still* contain natural toxins. Even today, cultures that eat large amounts of nightshades—like India, Brazil, and Indonesia—also have some of the highest cases of leprosy. Coincidence? Maybe. Maybe not. While leprosy itself is caused by bacteria, it's worth questioning whether some of those cases are actually solanine poisoning misdiagnosed as leprosy.

The real takeaway here is this: *Don't be a peasant.* Don't blindly accept the food narrative you've been spoon-fed since birth. If history teaches us anything, it's that people are *easily* manipulated into eating whatever benefits those in power. Just because something is edible doesn't mean it's optimal. And just because you've been told something is healthy doesn't mean it won't slowly wreck your body over time.

The question isn't just *what* you're eating—it's *who* convinced you to eat it in the first place.

And speaking of who, if you want to understand how deeply our food beliefs have been shaped by power, ego, and manipulation—not just with potatoes, but with entire dietary frameworks—you need to meet the man who changed the way America eats: Ancel Keys.

THE ANCEL KEYS DISASTER

The story of Ancel Keys and the food pyramid is a master class in how bad science, ego, and cherry-picked data can reshape an entire population's health—and not in a good way.

Let's start with who he was. Ancel Keys was a physiologist at the University of Michigan, obsessed with the idea that diet influenced health outcomes. Before he became infamous for his war on fat, he gained recognition for his Starvation Study—a brutal experiment where he deliberately starved men (mostly those unfit for war) to observe the physiological effects of prolonged caloric deprivation. It was grueling, but it put Keys on the map, setting the stage for his next big moment.

Fast forward to the 1950s when heart disease had become a national crisis. President Dwight Eisenhower suffered a heart attack and suddenly, America was desperate for answers. Keys saw his opportunity. He launched the Seven Countries Study, traveling across the world to collect dietary and health data. But instead of presenting his findings objectively, he cherry-picked data to fit his hypothesis: that dietary fat—especially saturated fat—was the primary driver of heart disease.

But guess what? *The full dataset didn't support his claims.* Countries like France, where butter and animal fats were dietary staples, had some of the lowest rates of heart disease. Instead of acknowledging the complexity of the issue, Keys simply ignored the data that didn't fit and published a wildly misleading conclusion.

He essentially invented cherry-picking data and crowned himself its godfather.

With his manipulated findings in hand, Keys convinced the US government to reshape its dietary recommendations, which resulted in the infamous and god-awful food pyramid. You know the one. The one that villainized fat and protein while promoting grains, fruits, and vegetables as the foundation of a "healthy" diet.

Keys cited the Mediterranean diet as proof of his theory, but the asshole completely misrepresented what Mediterranean cultures *actually* ate. They weren't living off olive oil and vegetables. Traditional Mediterranean diets were rich in lamb, fish, goat, and eggs. But that didn't fit his anti-fat agenda, so he left those details out.

Even worse, while Keys was busy demonizing butter and meat, he completely ignored the *real* culprits of heart disease—like processed foods loaded with hydrogenated oils. People weren't cooking with lard anymore; they were deep-frying everything in Crisco and seed oils. Add to that the chain-smoking epidemic—Eisenhower himself reportedly smoked four packs a day—and you start to see how absurdly narrow Keys's focus was. But instead of addressing these glaring health risks, the government doubled down on grains, grains, and more grains.

What. The. Fuck.

Was this an agenda to cripple human health? Or just a case of an arrogant scientist unwilling to admit he was wrong? Either way, the damage was done. Western medicine still clings to Keys's dietary dogma, and as a result, we're fatter, sicker, and drowning in chronic disease.

Keys missed the forest for the trees, and we're still suffering the consequences.

FROM THE FOOD PYRAMID TO MYPLATE: SAME SHIT, DIFFERENT TOILET

After decades of backlash against the food pyramid, the government tried to clean up its image with MyPlate—a new "personalized" approach to nutrition. The idea was to make healthy eating easier by dividing food into five categories: fruits, vegetables, grains, protein, and dairy. Vegetables and grains took up the largest portion, while protein got a measly little slice.

At first glance, MyPlate seems like an improvement, but when you break down the numbers, it's still a shitshow. A standard 2,400-calorie diet recommends just 6½ ounces of protein a day—which barely amounts to 40 grams of protein for a full-grown adult. Meanwhile, it pushes 3 cups of dairy and enough grains to equal eight slices of bread a day.

Let's just pause for a second. Eight slices of bread a day? Where in nature would you have stumbled upon the equivalent of that? There's no scenario fifteen thousand years ago where you'd find eight ounces of oatmeal and three cups of vegetables in a single day. It's an artificial construct, based on artificially abundant food.

Also, 3 cups of vegetables? Where are these measurements coming from? Somewhere along the way, we got tricked into measuring and micromanaging every bite of food we eat. People these days weigh their chicken breast to the gram, track their macros, and think that hitting an exact serving of fruits and vegetables will somehow guarantee health. But measuring food is an unnatural and modern construct. It's certainly not how our ancestors ate.

No hunter-gatherer was walking around with a food scale, making sure they had exactly 3½ ounces of protein before moving on with their day. They ate what was available, and availability changed constantly. Some days were feasts, some were famine. Some seasons were abundant, others required long periods of scarcity.

Modern nutrition guidance tells you to eat the same way, every day—same calories, same meals, same portion sizes. But nature doesn't work that way. Everything in nature is seasonal, unpredictable, and varied—and that's what kept our ancestors strong. Even intermittent fasting, while a step in the right direction, often turns into just another rigid schedule divorced from nature.

While the shift from the food pyramid to MyPlate was an attempt to "fix" public skepticism, it's still based on a broken paradigm. Grains and dairy weren't what fueled strong civilizations—meat was. And yet, we've been force-fed this idea that the foods propping up modern agriculture are those that should be propping up our health.

MY GRANDPARENTS ARE ROLLING IN THEIR GRAVES

The way we eat today didn't happen by accident. It wasn't just one bad decision—it was a slow unraveling, a series of choices made out of desperation, greed, and, in some cases, pure ignorance.

It started with *efficiency*. The Industrial Revolution cranked food production into overdrive. Factories took over, refining and processing foods to last longer, ship farther, and feed more people with less effort.

Then came *survival*. When the Great Depression hit in 1929, it wiped out millions of family farms and ranches. People didn't have a choice—they had to eat whatever was cheap, shelf-stable, and easy to mass-produce. Meat was expensive. Fresh food was scarce. So they turned to grains, potatoes, and processed foods—whatever would fill their stomachs and keep them from starving.

The goal wasn't health; it was not dying.

I grew up hearing those stories firsthand. Back home in Forks, Washington, my family ran a ranch. We didn't grow corn or grains; we raised cattle. It was a small town, with maybe five or six other ranches nearby, but these ranchers fed the town. Community members would buy whole cows or half cows, stocking their freezers for the year because they didn't have the land to raise their own.

But during the Depression, ranches like ours were wiped out. Nearly 750,000 family ranches disappeared through foreclosure or bankruptcy. When the ranches disappeared, so did the meat. People turned to survival foods—grains, potatoes, canned goods, and processed products from the Industrial Revolution. My grandparents never glorified those foods. They didn't romanticize bread and potatoes. They didn't think oatmeal was some kind of superfood. They saw those foods for what they were: *desperation meals*.

The Depression ended, but we never went back to the way we were eating before. Instead, we doubled down. We took industrialized food production and scaled it even further, refining, modifying, and manufacturing foods into something that looked like food but didn't act like it. Instead of returning to real food, we embraced lab-made convenience, prioritizing shelf life over nutrients and profit over health.

No matter how advanced we became, one thing never changed: *nature still makes the rules.* When we follow them, we thrive. When we don't, we pay the price.

Even when things seem natural, they often aren't. We've been manipulating plants for thousands of years, selectively breeding them to suit our tastes. Walk through the Midwest today, and you'll see endless fields of corn—corn that doesn't belong there. Wild corn would never survive in Wisconsin, yet we've forced it into existence, disrupting ecosystems just to fuel our food system.

And then came the final blow. Ancel Keys entered the scene, pushing the idea that fat and meat were the enemies, while bread and grains were the answer. The Mediterranean diet made olive oil and pasta look sexy, and suddenly, we had a whole generation thinking that a plate full of bread was somehow healthier than a steak.

My grandparents would be rolling in their graves if they knew we were putting bread and potatoes above meat.

THE MOST OUTRAGEOUS LIE

Thanks to the Industrial Revolution, assholes like Ancel Keys, and the stupid-ass food pyramid, we all grew up believing we were omnivores. That we *needed* plants. That we *had* to eat our vegetables. That a "balanced diet" meant piling greens on our plate like good little herbivores. But that's the biggest, most outrageous fucking lie we've ever been sold.

We are, and always have been, carnivores.

Humans don't need plants to thrive. We never did. We've just been brainwashed into thinking we do. And if you don't believe me—even after everything you've read so far—the proof is in our digestive systems, right in our stomach acid.

Stomach acid is measured on a pH scale from 0 to 14, with lower numbers being more acidic. The more acidic your stomach, the better it is at digesting meat and breaking down pathogens.

For example, white-backed vultures—pure scavengers that eat *rotting* meat—have a stomach pH of 1.2. The stomach acid in their digestive tracts is hyperacidic in order to kill bacteria. Opossums, another scavenger species, have a stomach pH of 1.5.

Guess where our stomach acid lies? Right there with the opossums, at 1.5.

For comparison, cats—textbook carnivores—have a pH of 3.6. Dogs sit at 4.5.

So let's get this straight: we're told we evolved from fruit- and leaf-munching primates, yet our stomach acid is far more carnivorous than theirs? Our digestive system is designed to tear through meat, fat, and pathogens just like a scavenger, yet somehow we're supposed to believe that fruits, veggies, and grains should be the foundation of our diet?

That's the lie.

And it's not just stomach acid. The structure of our entire digestive system screams meat-eater. Check it out:

1. **Our colons are short.** Herbivores like cows have massive colons because they need long fermentation times to break down fibrous plants. Humans don't have that. We have small colons and highly acidic stomachs—optimized for digesting animal protein, not grass and grains.
2. **Our intestines prioritize fat absorption.** Carnivores thrive on fat. Humans thrive on fat too. Our intestines are built to absorb fatty acids efficiently—something you don't see in pure herbivores.
3. **We lack the enzymes to break down plant toxins effectively.** Herbivores have the ability to detoxify plant defenses. We don't. That's why people struggle with oxalates, lectins, and nightshades—our bodies weren't built to process them.

We are not omnivores—and we never were.

NOMADIC WISDOM: EATING LIKE A HUMAN SHOULD

If we want to cut through the bullshit and find out what actually supports human health, we need to look at the people who never lost that connection: traditional nomadic tribes—the ones who live outside, move with the land, and don't need a nutrition degree to know what food is. Because when you strip away the modern noise, when you look at the people who still live in harmony with nature, the lesson is crystal clear: *they eat mostly meat.*

They're not foraging for kale or blending up antioxidant-rich açai bowls. They're not obsessing over whether their macros are balanced or if they're getting enough fiber. They don't wake up debating whether they should go keto, paleo, or vegan. They don't *diet*—they simply eat. They eat what their environment provides.

And what does nature provide? Animals.

Look at the Inuit. The Maasai. The Mongols. The Hadza. The Nenets. The Sami. The Gauchos. These tribes and cultures, despite being spread across different continents, have one thing in common: their diets are centered around eating other animals.

The Inuit, living in the Arctic, don't have grocery stores. They don't have year-round access to plants or fresh fruits. They eat whale, seal, caribou, and fish. They thrive in one of the harshest environments on Earth eating almost *exclusively* animal products.

The Maasai of Africa drink raw milk and blood from their cattle. The Mongols, the fierce warriors who conquered half the known world, lived on a diet of fermented horse milk and animal meat. The Hadza, one of the last true hunter-gatherer tribes, prioritize hunting over gathering—they don't waste time picking through the forest for a handful of berries when they could kill an animal that will sustain them for weeks.

For these nomadic tribes, their way of life isn't about preference. It's not about convenience either. It's about living optimally. Meat is strength. Meat is king. Meat is what builds strong bodies, sharp minds, and powerful, resilient people.

Contrast that with the modern world, where we've been convinced that eating a plate full of quinoa, tofu, and soy milk is somehow superior. That stuffing ourselves with grains, seed oils, and lab-grown meat is the future of health. That we should fear red meat while slathering plant-based butter (made from industrial chemicals) on our toast.

We have it completely fucking backward.

The people who still live in sync with nature are stronger, healthier, and more resilient than the average modern human. They don't suffer from the diseases that plague us. Their teeth are straight, their bones are strong, and their bodies function the way they're supposed to. They are living proof that when we eat what we were built to eat, *we thrive.*

Their way of life is a reminder of what we've lost and what we need to reclaim. They're connected to the land, to the animals they hunt, to the natural cycles that dictate their lives. They respect the balance of nature. They know that food isn't about indulgence or emotional comfort (more on this in the next chapter)—it's about *fueling the body in the most effective way possible.*

Nature has been telling us what we need to thrive all along.

And if you're the type who rolls your eyes at anecdotal evidence and needs cold, hard studies to believe something—don't worry, I've got you, girlfriend. Allow me to introduce to you Weston A. Price.

Price, a Canadian dentist and researcher in the early twentieth century, spent decades studying the relationship between diet and health. He traveled the world examining indigenous and isolated societies, documenting how traditional diets—rich in nutrient-dense, unprocessed animal foods—produced people with strong physiques, excellent dental health, and resistance to modern diseases. His findings were later compiled in his groundbreaking book, *Nutrition and Physical Degeneration.*

Price observed that as soon as these societies transitioned to Western diets high in processed grains, sugar, and industrialized foods, their health rapidly declined. Cavities, deformities, weakened immune systems, and chronic illnesses became widespread. Meanwhile, the societies that continued eating the way their ancestors did—consuming real, whole, animal-based foods—remained strong, healthy, and free from modern disease well into old age.

It's not a mystery—*meat builds strength and plants don't.* The evidence was clear in Price's research, just as it was in history. Societies that depended heavily on grains, like the peasants of medieval Europe, were shorter, weaker, and riddled with disease, while those who maintained ancestral diets flourished.

And yet, here we are today, acting like we've learned nothing. People are still being sold the idea that fruits, vegetables, and grains should be the foundation of their diet. They see these vegan influencers on Instagram with their perfectly curated smoothie bowls and raw salads, and they think, *That's what health looks like.*

But it's a scam—nothing could be further from the truth.

And since we're already talking about bullshit, let's moo-ve on to one of the dumbest arguments the plant-pushing crowds love to make.

WE ARE NOT COWS

One of the dumbest arguments floating around in vegan circles is, "Cows get their protein from plants, so why can't we?"

Let's break this down and educate the fools.

Cows don't magically extract protein from grass. They have an entire internal fermentation system—an ecosystem of specialized gut bacteria—that does the heavy lifting for them. *They* don't digest the grass. The bacteria inside them do. And then, the cows *get their nutrition from ingesting the bacteria.*

Cows are ruminants, meaning their digestive system is completely different from ours. Their stomach is a four-part fermentation factory designed to break down fibrous plant material and convert it into essential fatty acids the cow can use as fuel. The microbes also sacrifice their lives to the cow, providing it with protein.

Here's how it works:

1. **The Rumen** (the largest compartment) is a giant fermentation vat. Cows graze all day, swallowing food mostly unchewed. The rumen is filled with billions of microbes—bacteria, protozoa, and fungi—whose sole job is to break down tough plant fibers into usable compounds.
2. **The Reticulum** traps large, undigested particles and sends them back up the esophagus to be chewed again. This is called **rumination**, or cud-chewing. Cows spend hours each day doing this—breaking down plant material over and over to make it digestible.
3. **The Omasum** acts as a filter, removing excess water and further grinding down the plant material before sending it along.
4. **The Abomasum** is the closest thing to a human stomach, where digestive acids break down whatever remains before the real absorption happens.

In other words: *Cows don't survive on grass. They survive on the protein and fatty acids produced by the bacteria in their stomachs.*

The bacteria eat the grass. The bacteria multiply. Then, when those bacteria die, the cow digests *them* for protein. That's where the real nutrition comes from—not the grass itself, but the microbial byproducts and dead bacteria that get absorbed later in the digestive process.

As such, cows are technically *bacterial carnivores*. They have a built-in fermentation system that lets them survive on plant material—but what they're actually absorbing isn't the grass itself. It's the *fatty acids* and *microbial proteins* created during the fermentation process.

So no, you *cannot* get your protein the same way cows do. You don't have a built-in fermentation chamber. You don't have a reticulum to chew your food twice. You don't have a microbiome designed to turn grass into fatty acids.

You are not a cow.

WHY CORN-FED COWS GET SICK

When I was a kid, my grandpa would always say, "You can't feed cows corn; it'll make them sick." He was right. Feeding cows grains is a disaster.

Corn, which has been so genetically manipulated it barely resembles its wild counterpart, is one of the biggest clown foods out there. Feeding it to cows promotes harmful bacterial growth, compromises their health, and ultimately degrades the quality of the meat and milk they produce. It's a stark contrast to cows raised on their natural diet of grass and herbs, which support the right kind of bacteria and keep the cow thriving.

Grain-fed cows develop acidosis (an overproduction of acid in the rumen), which leads to infections, inflammation, and immune system breakdown. This is why factory-farmed cows are pumped full of antibiotics—not to keep them "healthy," but to keep them alive long enough to fatten them up for slaughter.

And if you think that *doesn't* affect you, think again.

The meat from grain-fed cows has a totally different nutritional profile than that of grass-fed cows. When cows eat grass, their meat is rich in omega-3 fatty acids, CLA (conjugated linoleic acid), and vitamin K2—all essential for human health. In contrast, meat from grain-fed cows is inflamed and loaded with omega-6 fatty acids, which drive inflammation and disease.

This is why eating high-quality meat from properly raised animals matters. A healthy cow produces nutrient-dense meat that fuels human health. A sick, grain-fed, antibiotic-riddled cow produces garbage meat that fuels metabolic disease.

In nature, everything works in harmony. When you disrupt that harmony—whether with genetically altered foods, artificial feeding practices, or antibiotics—you're not just messing with cows, you're messing with the entire system that supports them—and by extension, us.

So why does this matter to you? Because the same logic applies to *your* diet.

A cow fed the wrong diet gets sick. A human fed the wrong diet gets sick too. Cows weren't built to eat grains. Humans weren't built to eat grains either. Cows need bacteria to ferment plants into usable nutrition. *We do not.* Our digestive system is not designed to turn plants into protein.

If you think you can live off plants just because a cow does, you're not just misinformed, you're proving exactly how easy it is to control and manipulate people with bad science. The same people who pushed the food pyramid, who told you to fear fat, are the ones who convinced you that fruits and vegetables are essential. They're not.

WHAT TO EAT: THE HIERARCHY OF ANIMAL FOODS

You made it to the part of the chapter that talks about what to eat. Finally! And the answer is simple, but nuanced. So what should we actually be eating? Meat—no surprises there.

But not just any meat—the right kinds, in the right order. Here they are:

1. **Ruminant animals (the gold standard):** Ruminants—like cows, bison, elk, lamb, and deer—are the most nutrient-dense, easily digestible protein sources for humans. Their digestive system breaks down plant matter for us, converting it into high-quality protein, fat, and essential micronutrients like B12, heme iron, zinc, and conjugated linoleic acid (CLA). If you want strength, longevity, and metabolic health, ruminant meat should be the foundation of your diet.

2. **Fish (especially cold-water fish):** After ruminants, wild-caught, cold-water fish—like salmon, sardines, mackerel, herring, and anchovies—are the next-best option. They provide essential omega-3 fatty acids (EPA and DHA), which support brain function, reduce inflammation, and balance the omega-6 overload from modern diets. The key is choosing fish low in toxins and heavy metals while being high in healthy fats.

3. **Poultry (good, but not the best):** Chicken and turkey are decent protein sources, but they lack the nutrient density of ruminant animals and fish. They're also higher in omega-6 fatty acids, which, when overconsumed, can contribute to inflammation—especially if the birds are fed a grain-based diet. If you eat poultry, opt for pasture-raised.

4. **Pork (eat it least):** Pork is biologically closer to human tissue than any other meat, which might sound cool until you realize that it also means our bodies recognize pork proteins differently. Studies suggest that pork can trigger more inflammation in some people compared to beef, lamb, or fish. The reason behind this is because pigs, like humans, are monogastric animals, meaning they don't have a specialized digestive system like ruminants to filter out toxins and refine nutrients. Their fat profile is also higher in inflammatory omega-6 fats, especially when they're fed grains. If you enjoy pork, eat it sparingly and choose pasture-raised over conventional grain-fed pork.

If you want to get sexy, you need to eat what your body was meant to eat. Eat like a queen, not a peasant. The closer your diet aligns with human physiology, the stronger, healthier, and sexier you'll be.

REINTRODUCING MICROBES: WHY FERMENTED FOODS MATTER

We've established that the proper human diet is meat. That's what our bodies are built for, what our ancestors thrived on, and what nomadic tribes still rely on today. But unfortunately, we don't live like our ancestors anymore.

For most of human history, we were constantly exposed to healthy microbes. We lived outside, walked barefoot on the earth, drank from natural water sources, hunted and butchered animals with our bare hands, and lived in tight-knit communities where bacteria were shared and passed around naturally. Our immune systems were constantly interacting with the environment, strengthening themselves, and adapting.

These days, unfortunately, we're sterilized to death.

We walk on pavement, wear shoes everywhere, bathe in chlorinated water, scrub our hands with antibacterial soap, and live in artificially controlled indoor environments. We're no longer rolling in the dirt, touching raw animal flesh daily, or drinking from rivers rich with beneficial bacteria—all of which has left our microbiome completely wrecked.

Your gut bacteria—the trillions of microbes that live inside you—play a massive role in your overall health. They influence digestion, immunity, hormone balance, and even mental clarity. In a natural world, we'd be replenishing these microbes every day simply by existing in nature. Since we don't live that way anymore, we have to be intentional about bringing those microbes back in.

And that's where fermented foods come in.

Fermented foods are the next-best thing to rolling around in the dirt and eating freshly killed meat. They're packed with beneficial bacteria that help restore balance to the gut, support digestion, and strengthen the immune system. Traditional cultures around the world have always included some form of fermented food in their diets—because before refrigeration, fermentation was how people preserved food.

Think about it. The Mongols drank fermented mare's milk (kumis). The Japanese eat fermented soybeans (natto). Koreans have kimchi. Germans have sauerkraut. Eastern Europeans have kvass. Every culture had some version of fermented foods because they understood—whether consciously or not—that these foods supported digestion and overall health.

So if you want to thrive in today's world—where everything is too clean, too controlled, and too removed from nature—you need to add fermented foods back into your diet.

The simplest way to do this is to include traditional fermented foods in your daily routine. Things like:

- **Raw sauerkraut:** Not the vinegar-soaked stuff from the grocery store, but real, fermented cabbage teeming with live probiotics.
- **Kimchi:** Spicy, fermented Korean cabbage that's loaded with beneficial bacteria.
- **Kefir:** A fermented dairy drink with significantly more probiotics than yogurt.
- **Yogurt:** But only if it's raw, full-fat, and fermented properly. None of that sugary, low-fat crap.
- **Raw cheese:** Aged, unpasteurized cheese is rich in good bacteria.

These foods are the missing piece in the modern diet. They help repopulate the gut with beneficial bacteria, making up for what we've lost by living in an overly sanitized world. While meat gives you your body's fuel, fermented foods give you the gut strength to absorb it properly. It's not the vegetables themselves—it's the microbes living on them that matter.

THE SIMPLEST PATH TO REAL HEALTH

The modern food system has turned us into lab rats, feeding us clown food that's been stripped, manipulated, and engineered beyond recognition. From selectively bred plants overloaded with sugar to grain-fed livestock pumped full of antibiotics, we've been tricked into believing we're eating real food when we're not.

But nature never changed the principles—only humans did.

If you want to reclaim your vitality, the answer is simple: ditch the clown food and nourish your body with what it's meant to eat. That means real, unprocessed meat, nutrient-dense animal foods, and fermented staples that restore the gut.

The closer you eat to nature, the stronger, healthier, and sexier you'll become.

PRINCIPLE #3

FIND JOY OUTSIDE OF FOOD

"I could never live without bread—it makes me so happy!"
"What's the point of life if I can't enjoy a bowl of pasta?"
"Giving up sugar would make me miserable."
"Ice cream is my therapy."
"I don't drink, I don't smoke—just let me have my damn cookies!"
"Food is the only joy I have left."

Look at those statements. Really look at them. These are real statements I've heard from women throughout the years. How sad is it that we've been conditioned to believe that true happiness—actual joy—comes from bread, a bowl of pasta, or a scoop of ice cream?

That last one especially—*food is the only joy I have left*. That's not just sad; that's fucking terrifying. Because if that's true, then what does that say about the rest of your life?

In this chapter, I'm going to dismantle these lies. I'll break down the difference between joy and pleasure—why one lasts and the other fades the second you swallow. We'll talk about how real joy isn't found in comfort, but in adversity. You'll learn why food is fuel, not an emotional crutch, and how changing the way you eat will change your mood, your mindset, and your resilience. You'll also see how the world tries to pull you out of your frame, how to stand your ground, and why sometimes, a little shame is exactly what's needed to snap you out of a destructive cycle.

JOY VS. PLEASURE: UNDERSTANDING THE DIFFERENCE

At the core of human experience, happiness comes from two sources: joy and pleasure. Everything we associate with "happiness" falls into one of these two categories. But if you want real fulfillment—and if you want to break free from destructive food habits—you have to understand the difference between them.

Pleasure is sensory. It's fleeting. It's tied to taste, touch, sound, sight, or smell. It's the dopamine rush when you bite into a perfectly seared ribeye or run your fingers over soft fur. It's fun, instant, and everywhere—the first sip of a drink, the crisp sound of a vinyl record spinning, the warmth of a fresh blanket out of the dryer. Even sex, for all its intimacy, often falls into this category. Because it's not the act itself that brings joy—it's the bond it creates.

Joy, on the other hand, is deeper. It lingers. It's love, gratitude, and connection—the things that make life meaningful. Listening to *Dark Side of the Moon* in your car? That's pleasure. Seeing Pink Floyd live, surrounded by thousands of people, all feeling the same magic? That's joy.

Pleasure fades the moment it's over. Joy stays with you. It changes you. It becomes part of who you are.

FOOD IS NEVER JOY

Unfortunately, we've been programmed to believe that pleasure and joy are the same thing—especially when it comes to food.

How many times have you heard someone say, "That homemade sourdough brings me so much joy," or "This ice cream is pure joy"? But that's not joy. That's just pleasure.

That pasta, that croissant, that perfectly cooked steak—it's lighting up your brain the same way a hit of nicotine or a slot machine payout would. It's not happiness. It's a biological trick, a primal survival mechanism designed to make us crave energy-dense foods when they were scarce. Except today, food isn't scarce. And that mechanism has turned against us.

For most of human history, our ancestors got 95 to 98 percent of their calories from meat. Finding honey or a berry bush was rare, and our brains developed a strong dopamine response to sugar because it meant survival. Sugar wasn't supposed to be easy to get—it was supposed to be a jackpot.

But now, the ratio is flipped. Instead of 98 percent meat and 2 percent sugar, modern diets are 80 percent sugar and carbs, with maybe 20 percent coming from real food. And because our brains are still wired to treat sugar like a rare treasure, we've built an entire culture that chases pleasure at the expense of joy.

And that's exactly how the food industry wants it.

The food industry has made it its mission to convince us that food *is* happiness. That a cookie is love. That a slice of cake is celebration. That a bowl of pasta is comfort. They've spent billions tying food to connection, nostalgia, and belonging. And we've swallowed the lie whole.

Think about it: Is it the turkey that makes Thanksgiving special? Or is it the people at the table? Would your grandmother's cookies still hold meaning if they were store-bought? Of course not. Because it was never about the food—it was about the love, the memory, the experience.

Food is just the medium. It's what happens *while* joy is unfolding, not the joy itself.

But the food industry doesn't want you to see that. They want you to believe a cupcake can bring you happiness when all it really does is light up your brain for five minutes before leaving you wanting more. Because the moment you recognize the difference between pleasure and joy, they lose their grip on you.

And once you see the lie, you can't unsee it.

You start recognizing just how much time you've spent chasing pleasure instead of building joy. You realize that the dopamine hit from sugar, carbs, and hyperpalatable foods isn't real happiness—it's just a chemical trick designed to keep you coming back for more.

And the moment you stop looking to food to make you happy—when you stop saying, "I need this treat to celebrate" or "I deserve this because I had a hard day"—that's when you get your power back. Because true joy never comes from a plate.

It comes from how you live your life.

FOOD IS FUEL AND INFORMATION

Thanks to the food industry's marketing, we've forgotten what food actually is. We've turned it into comfort, entertainment, and emotional support. We treat it like a reward system instead of a survival tool.

But food isn't therapy—it's fuel.

And not just because it powers your body, but because it programs it. Like we said in Chapter 1: food is information. Every bite sends instructions to your DNA—flipping genetic switches that influence everything from metabolism to fertility to longevity. What you eat doesn't just affect you now—it echoes for generations.

So when you fuel yourself with garbage, you don't just feel like garbage. You *become* it—bloated, sluggish, foggy, and constantly battling cravings. But when you eat like a human is meant to, you feel strong, clear, energized, grounded, and sexy AF.

Unfortunately, most people treat their bodies like they're disposable. They shovel in processed grains, sugar, and empty carbs like it's no big deal—then wonder why they're inflamed, exhausted, and always chasing the next hit.

But let's get one thing straight: your body isn't a junker. It's a high-performance machine designed for strength, speed, and precision. Unfortunately, most people are out there pouring cheap, watered-down fuel into it, then acting surprised when the engine sputters.

If you actually owned a fancy race car, you wouldn't pump it full of low-grade gas. You'd give it premium fuel—because that's what it was built for. Your body is no different. It was designed to run on meat that comes from nature. And deep down, you know that. Strip away the noise—the grocery stores, the marketing, the convenience—and your instincts kick in. That's why the smell of a steak sizzling on the grill makes your mouth water. That's why a trout fried in a cast-iron pan hits differently. Your body knows it's the proper fuel.

Now compare that to eggplant parmesan. Or a pile of steamed cauliflower. Or a big Caesar salad with croutons. Did your mouth water at all?

I didn't think so.

Stop eating for fun and start eating for function. Stop relying on food to fix your feelings. Stop being owned by cravings, impulses, and the idea that food should *make you happy.* The second you stop pretending food is your friend, your therapist, or your entertainment, you'll get your joy back.

HOW ADDICTION DULLS JOY

When you chase too much pleasure, it starts to dull your ability to feel joy. This is how addiction works—whether it's sugar, alcohol, drugs, you name it. The endless pursuit of pleasure *at the expense of everything else* rewires your brain, making it harder and harder to experience real happiness.

In other words, the more pleasure you chase, the more joy gets drowned out.

Breaking that cycle means removing the overload of pleasure. It's not easy. The brain's pleasure pathways need time to heal and recalibrate. But when you strip away the artificial highs—the processed foods, the sugar, the quick hits—you create space for joy to reemerge.

It's like going blind and realizing your other senses have become sharper. Deprive yourself of fleeting pleasures, and suddenly, you'll feel the depth of joy again. Not because you forced it, but because you finally made room for it.

THE MOMENTS THAT ACTUALLY MATTER

For me, it all clicked one night when I was lying in bed, staring at the ceiling, asking myself what I'd take with me when it's all said and done. What will I remember when I'm 120 and the noise of life has gone quiet?

It won't be the steak, even though you know I love a good one. It won't be the vacations, the shoes, or the stuff. It's not even the body I've worked so damn hard for. None of that comes with you.

What I'll remember are the nights I held my boys as they fell asleep with their little fingers tangled in my hair, their warm little breaths on my neck. I'll remember how tight Tom held my hand while I read him my wedding vows. I'll remember sitting with my mom and sister on the porch during summer, the way my dad smelled after a long day of fishing on the river, and slumber parties with my childhood girlfriends. I'll remember moments of silence in nature so thick they felt holy.

Those are the moments that make life full. Not the cheap highs, not the dopamine hits. Just real connection, deep presence, and love. That's what stays.

And when I realized that—when I *really* felt that in my bones—I stopped pretending that food was anything more than fuel. The joy isn't in the chocolate. It's in the life I'm trying to be awake for.

TOM'S TAKE: CHASING THE WRONG THINGS

Everything changed for me when I came across a book called *The Happiness Formula*. It laid out this simple truth: happiness comes from either joy or pleasure. That's it. I remember closing the book and just sitting there thinking, *Well, damn*. That wasn't just an insight—it was a complete mindset shift.

Before that, I was chasing pleasure without even realizing it. Food, drinks, distractions—whatever gave me that quick hit of dopamine. But once I understood the difference, I started making different choices. I stopped mistaking fleeting pleasure for something deeper.

Joy, I realized, was almost always tied to connection. The moments that stand out in my life aren't the ones where I got what I wanted or bought something cool—they're the ones where I felt fully present. Laughing with Candi until we couldn't breathe. Watching my kids do something brave or surprising. Sitting around a fire, not needing to say much, just enjoying the warmth, the stillness, the company.

Joy doesn't need to be loud. It's not performative. It's not complicated.

Now don't get me wrong, I still enjoy pleasures—cars, good food, and new gadgets—but I don't pretend those things are what make life meaningful. I also find pleasure in competition, in chaos, in the thrill of new ideas. Joy, to me these days, is thinking about ways to grow our business, how we can help people, spinning fresh concepts into something tangible—it's exciting, and it keeps my mind moving.

What I'm after now is a life that feels real. One built on connection, on presence, on purpose. And the more I lean into that, the less I need anything else.

THE ROLE OF ADVERSITY IN FINDING JOY

After reflecting on what truly matters—on what actually brings lasting happiness—you start to see the pattern. The moments that mean something, the ones that stay with you, almost always come with a little struggle. They're not handed to you. They're earned.

Those struggles didn't just make life harder—*they made life meaningful.*

But modern life has stripped that away. We wake up in temperature-controlled homes, drive in air-conditioned cars, and spend our days in artificial comfort. If we're hungry, we tap an app. If we're cold, we turn a dial. Everything is optimized for ease. Struggle has become something we outsource, avoid, or medicate away.

And yet, something's missing. Because we aren't designed for comfort. We're designed for *challenge*.

Humans are problem-solvers by nature. We're built to overcome obstacles, to adapt, to fight for survival. When survival isn't on the table, however, we start creating problems where there aren't any.

Without real adversity, we invent stupid-ass problems.

We stress over trivial shit—like whether or not we should eat a bowl of ice cream—as if it's some profound internal battle. Past generations fought wars, endured plagues, and survived famines while we're over here acting like choosing between oat milk or almond milk is a life-altering decision.

Your problem isn't your ice cream addiction.

Your problem is that you don't have real fucking problems.

We've become spoiled brats, expecting all the rewards with none of the effort. We chase dopamine through food, entertainment, and social media, but those hits are empty. They don't satisfy. They don't mean anything. Real joy? It comes from doing hard things. From overcoming. From earning it.

If you want more joy, stop running from adversity and instead, start choosing it.

HOW TO SIMULATE ADVERSITY IN A SOFT WORLD

The modern world doesn't challenge us naturally, so we have to manufacture our own adversity. And no, that doesn't mean making your life harder for no reason. It means reintroducing the challenges that shaped us into strong, capable humans.

Here are a few ways to do that:

1. **Fasting:** Our ancestors didn't eat three meals a day. They didn't have snack drawers or convenience stores. Some days, the hunt failed and they went without food. That was normal. Fasting isn't a diet trend—it's a way to mimic the natural cycles of feast and famine that kept humans strong. Skipping a meal won't kill you, but it will retrain your brain to stop expecting instant gratification.

2. **Cold exposure:** Imagine waking up in the wild on a freezing morning with no heater. That's the reality our ancestors faced *every day*. Cold therapy—whether through cold showers, winter hikes, or ice plunges—triggers primal survival instincts that modern life has numbed. It forces your body to adapt, toughens your mind, and leaves you feeling sharp and alive.

3. **Hard physical work:** Our ancestors didn't hit the gym. They sprinted to hunt. They carried heavy loads. They built things with their hands. Modern workouts have been sanitized—controlled, predictable, and safe. But real strength comes from moving the way humans were meant to: lifting heavy things, sprinting, climbing, carrying, and enduring.

4. **Aligning with nature's cycles:** Before artificial light, humans lived by the sun. They woke up with daylight, worked in harmony with the seasons, and rested when it was dark. Today, we fight those natural rhythms with screens, stimulants, and artificial schedules. The solution? Wake up with the sun. Spend more time outside and reduce artificial light at night (more on this in Chapters 5 and 6).

STAYING IN YOUR FRAME

When you start changing your life—whether it's how you eat, how you think, or how you treat your body—you will make other people uncomfortable. That's just the truth. Especially when you stop turning to food for joy, comfort, or connection. Most people don't know how to handle that, because most people rely on food for all those things. So when you start finding joy outside of cheesecake or wine nights, it threatens their entire worldview.

Here's where *staying in your frame* comes in.

The concept comes from a book Tom and I loved called *Pitch Anything*, and while it was written for sales and business, the core ideas apply perfectly here. Everyone walks around with their own "frame"—a mental lens that shapes how they see the world. The person with the stronger frame sets the tone of any interaction. When you don't know how to hold your frame, you'll constantly find yourself adapting to other people's opinions, emotions, and expectations—even if they contradict your own.

When you're on a healthy journey to get sexy, this shows up fast. You'll hear things like:

"Oh, come on, one bite won't kill you."

"You're being extreme."

"You don't need to lose weight—you already look great!"

These aren't neutral comments; they're subtle frame tests. And if you don't stay rooted in your own, you'll find yourself explaining, defending, or justifying something that doesn't need explaining.

It's not about being combative. It's about not abandoning yourself.

Staying in your frame means holding onto your purpose and your perspective, even when others push back. It means not shrinking to make other people more comfortable with your growth.

So for example, when someone says, "I could never give up carbs," you don't have to nod and say, "Yeah, it's hard." Instead, you can calmly reply, "That's because you're not ready yet." No judgment. No defense. Just the truth. Staying in your frame means you don't match someone else's energy.

Why does this matter? Because if you're always living in someone else's frame, you'll never feel rooted in your own. And if you're not rooted, you're easily shaken—second-guessing yourself, tiptoeing around other people's feelings, or hiding your progress to keep others comfortable. That's when sabotage creeps in.

I've seen this happen over and over in the Primal Bod community. A woman starts feeling amazing—energy high, sleep dialed in, weight dropping, libido back online—and then someone close to her makes a snarky comment. One little seed of doubt, and suddenly, she's spiraling.

She's not spiraling because she failed. It's because she left her frame.

I'm not saying you need to armor up and walk through life on the defensive. I'm saying you need to stay grounded. You don't need anyone's permission to get healthy. You don't owe anyone an explanation for why you're eating differently, moving your body, or feeling sexy again. You're allowed to want more—and that doesn't make you rude, selfish, or weird.

The longer you stay in your frame, the stronger it gets. And the stronger it gets, the less you'll feel the need to justify anything to anyone.

Here's a question I want you to sit with—and it may be one of the most important questions to ask yourself: Why do you care what sick people think?

I might not know your exact circle, but chances are, most of the people around you—friends, coworkers, even family—aren't healthy. Not physically. Not mentally. Not emotionally. So why let *them* shape your decisions? My mom used to say, "If everyone's jumping off a bridge, does that mean you need to?" Exactly.

So stay in your frame. You're not being extreme; you're following nature's principles.

IT'S TIME TO BRING SHAME BACK

If we're going to reclaim real health (and real joy), we have to bring back the tools that kept us strong. One of those tools is shame. And I'm not talking about the twisted, cancel-culture version that gets weaponized online. I'm talking about the kind of shame that held communities together. The kind that kept people accountable.

I've talked a lot about staying in your frame and not getting pulled into other people's excuses, but what happens when someone in your circle is actively dragging everyone down? That's where shame becomes useful. It's not about being cruel—it's about being real. Shame, when it's grounded in love, is a form of care, of love. It's how tribes kept their people in check. It's how we stop enabling bad behavior and start raising the bar—for ourselves *and* each other.

Somewhere along the way, society decided shame was always bad. That we should never use it because…*feelings*.

To which I say, *Fuck that*. It's time to bring shame back.

SHAME AS A SURVIVAL TOOL

In tribal societies, shame served an essential role. When someone behaved in a way that endangered the group—whether by laziness, selfishness, or outright stupidity—shame was the mechanism for course correction. It wasn't about cruelty; it was about survival. If one person's actions could jeopardize the group, they needed to be called out and held accountable. Shame was a form of feedback, a tool to ensure everyone pulled their weight and upheld their responsibilities.

Without shame, there's no accountability. Without accountability, the group falls apart.

Before diving deeper into the role of shame, it's important to first distinguish it from rejection. Rejection and shame often get lumped together, but they're not the same. Rejection is external—it's the tribe deciding you're no longer worth their resources or time. Shame, on the other hand, is internal. It forces you to confront your own behavior, to feel the sting of knowing you've let yourself and others down.

Now, most people would rather face rejection than shame. They'll leave a situation, walk away from relationships, or quit entirely just to avoid the discomfort of shame. But that's precisely why shame is so powerful. It's the last line of defense when all else fails. If someone refuses to take responsibility, refuses to feel remorse, shame is the only thing that can snap them out of their self-destructive cycle.

And that's why, in the end, *shame is kindness*.

It might sound counterintuitive, but shaming someone can be the kindest thing you ever do for them. It forces them to confront the truth. Shame, when wielded appropriately, isn't about cruelty or humiliation. It's about honesty. It's about saying, "This behavior is unacceptable, and it's hurting you and those around you."

Say a fat girl who wants to lose weight but constantly complains about it starts up again: "I just don't know why I can't lose weight," she says. Instead of stepping into her frame, nodding along, or offering sympathy, you look her straight in the eye and say, "Yeah, but you sure do love chocolate cake."

Blasphemy, right? Maybe you think that's inappropriate. Or rude. But if you strip away your conditioning, it's just the truth. When did telling someone they love cheesecake become offensive? Only when you're trapped in their frame. It's not an insult. It's a fact.

And if that fact makes them uncomfortable, *that discomfort is an opportunity for growth*—and that is a gift. Shame is the antidote to denial. It strips away the excuses, the justifications, and the victim mentality, leaving only the raw truth.

And from that place of truth, change becomes possible.

Of course, not all shame is created equal. To use it effectively—and to respond to it effectively—you need to evaluate the intent behind it. Are they shaming you out of malice, to tear you down and feed their own insecurities? Or are they coming from a place of care, trying to help you see what you're blind to?

This distinction matters.

THE MODERN MISUSE OF SHAME

There's a difference between constructive shame that pushes you toward growth and manipulative shame designed to control or belittle. The former is a gift; the latter is abuse. Learn to tell the difference.

In today's world, shame has been weaponized in the wrong way. Instead of encouraging personal accountability, it's used to enforce blanket acceptance of everything. Liberals shame conservatives for not being "progressive" enough. Corporations shame consumers into buying their "sustainable" products while raking in billions. It's a twisted, manipulative version of shame that serves no one but those in power.

True shame is grounded in truth. It's not about forcing people into ideological boxes or guilting them into compliance. It's about helping individuals recognize where they've gone astray so they can course-correct and thrive.

Avoiding shame is like avoiding adversity—it weakens you. Instead of running from it, embrace it. Let it show you where you need to grow, where you've been making excuses, and where you've been settling for less than your best.

Shame isn't your enemy; it's an opportunity to create joy.

So, the next time someone shames you, take a step back. Evaluate their intent. Are they trying to tear you down, or are they handing you the mirror you've been avoiding? If it's the latter, take a deep breath, swallow your pride, and do the hard work of change.

It might sting in the moment, but in the long run, it'll make you stronger, better, and more aligned with the person you want to be. I'm sure you can think of some moments right now. We all have them.

In fact, Tom and I are each going to share a time when shame helped us grow into better versions of ourselves.

HOW SHAME WOKE ME UP

One of the deepest moments of shame I've ever felt came after I left my first husband. He was paying $500 a month in child support for Shawn and Lane, while Robert's dad paid nothing. I was raising all three boys on my own—covering daycare, clothes, food, and everything else. That $500 barely made a dent.

I had agreed to the low amount out of guilt. My ex-husband didn't want the divorce, and I was trying to be "nice." Even my attorney said, "Why are you doing this? You're entitled to eight hundred dollars." But I didn't want conflict. I wanted peace.

After a year and a half of scraping by, I finally went back to court to ask for the $800 I should've gotten all along. I couldn't afford a lawyer, so I represented myself. I walked into that courtroom hopeful, a little desperate, and ready to make my case.

The judge didn't care. He looked at me and said, "Go find another job." He dismissed me, just like that. It was humiliating. I wasn't just embarrassed, I was ashamed. Ashamed that I had let myself rely on someone else. Ashamed that I had expected anyone to rescue me. Ashamed that I was sitting there, begging for $300 more a month like it would fix my life.

That moment lit a fire in me. I walked out of that courtroom and thought, *Never again.* I would never put myself in that position again. I wasn't going to beg, and I sure as hell wasn't going to depend on anyone else to provide for me or my kids.

I got to work.

At the time, I was a hairstylist, and I hustled like my life depended on it—because it did. I passed out business cards, raised my rates, worked weekends, and stayed late. Robert came to the salon with me in a bouncer. Shawn and Lane were the last kids picked up from daycare most nights. I was exhausted, but I made it work.

Was I scared? Absolutely. There were nights I laid awake thinking, *What have I done?* I was in a new town, with no support, raising three boys alone. But that courtroom humiliation turned out to be a gift. It showed me just how often I looked to other people to fix things I needed to face myself.

The shame I felt that day wasn't there to break me. It was a turning point. It pushed me to get clear, get organized, and figure things out in a way I never had before. Over time, it gave me a deeper sense of self-respect. I became more steady, more resourceful, and more confident in my ability to handle whatever came next.

TOM'S TAKE: THE POWER OF SHAME

I was shamed by a mentor once—and it was one of the most transformative experiences of my life. His name was Tom too—a guy about fifteen years older than me, incredibly successful, smart, and someone I really admired. At first, our relationship was professional, but over time, we became friends. One night at dinner, though, the gloves came off.

We sat down at the table, and he didn't waste any time. He started questioning everything—my life decisions, how I was managing my (first) marriage, how I was spending money. I remember feeling this wave of shame wash over me as he dug in.

"Why did you buy a BMW?" he asked.

"Well," I said, fumbling for words, "you gotta have fun when you're young, right? You might not make it to old age."

He just looked at me. "Do you really believe that? Because there's a 90-something percent chance you'll live to be seventy or eighty. So, do you really believe what you just said, or is that just a justification for your behavior?"

I didn't know what to say. I felt embarrassed—small, like a kid getting scolded for doing something stupid. And he had joked with me about this stuff before, but I hadn't listened. This time, though, I couldn't ignore it. His words hit me hard, and for the first time, I heard him.

I took a moment to evaluate his intent. He wasn't trying to tear me down. He wasn't being mean. He was trying to help me. And I realized then that all his nice, joking attempts to steer me in the right direction had failed because I wasn't ready to listen. But now I was. By rubbing my face in the truth, he forced me to confront it. It was uncomfortable, but it was exactly what I needed.

And let me tell you, I felt *so small*. You know that feeling when you suddenly realize you've been completely wrong about something? It's like your whole presence shrinks. At one point, as I was talking, I thought, *Do I sound like Mickey Mouse right now? Is my voice higher?*

But you know what? That's when I knew he'd gotten through to me. I didn't need to say anything else. I just needed to shut my mouth and listen.

That conversation stuck with me. Afterward, I began questioning myself—my justifications for spending money, the decisions I was making, even the beliefs I held about who I was and what I valued. Things I had thought were rock solid suddenly didn't seem so certain. It wasn't about being wrong or right anymore; it was about asking better questions.

I started to approach life differently. Instead of clinging to beliefs, I adopted a mindset of curiosity. Everything became a question. Even when I thought I was certain about something, I treated it as a hypothesis, not a fact. Living this way opened my eyes to the truth in a way I'd never experienced before.

That dinner didn't just change my perspective; it changed my life. It wasn't the first or last time I'd experience a moment like that, but it was one of the most pivotal. And it all started with someone I respected caring enough to shame me, to hold a mirror up to my face and force me to see what I was doing.

I wasn't angry with Tom for what he said to me. I wasn't upset, because I knew his intent was good. He cared enough to make me uncomfortable, to challenge me, and that's rare. Even my own parents, as much as they loved me, had failed to do that. They were trying to be "nice," and in doing so, they missed opportunities to help me grow into a stronger, better person.

Tom's tough love taught me one of the most important lessons of my life: shame, when used wisely, is kindness. It's a way of saying, "I care enough about you to call you out, to push you, to make you uncomfortable so you can grow."

To this day, I'm grateful for that dinner. It made me reevaluate my priorities and change the way I approached life. And it solidified my relationship with my mentor. He's still a great friend, one of the few people who've endured through the years. Why? Because I recognized that he wasn't trying to tear me down—he was building me up.

And that's what real care looks like.

RECLAIMING JOY, ONE CHOICE AT A TIME

When you strip away the distractions of fleeting pleasure, you create space for joy to thrive. That's the beauty of simplifying your life—of reconnecting with what actually matters. And it's not just about food. It's about breaking free from the illusion that pleasure equals happiness and reclaiming the joy that's been buried under years of dopamine-fueled conditioning.

So here's the challenge: Redefine your relationship with happiness. Recognize that food brings only pleasure, not joy. Understand that the constant pursuit of pleasure weakens your ability to feel real joy. And when you remove the noise—the sugar, the processed foods, the unnecessary indulgences—you can finally experience the raw, undiluted simplicity of life.

Joy resides in that simplicity.

This isn't a one-time fix. It's not a diet, a goal, or a box to check. It's a way of living—a mindset, a practice, and an ongoing effort. You don't just "get it" once and move on. You have to remind yourself daily. You have to recalibrate, recommit, and keep making choices that align with what truly matters.

Don't just change the way you eat; change the way you *think*. Stop letting food act as your shortcut to comfort, your substitute for connection, or your escape from modern- day stresses. Because in nature, food was always fuel first, not fulfillment. When you turn to food as your primary source of joy, you strip it away from its purpose. Our ancestors didn't find joy in bread baskets—they found it in movement, connection, challenge, and creation. Food was fuel, and joy came from living.

So let it be that for you too. Let food support your life—not *be* your life.

Because getting sexy is deeper than cutting carbs or fitting into your high school jeans (although you will feel sexy doing those things too!). It's about feeling vibrant, radiant, and connected again.

Your ancestors knew how to live like that.

Now it's your turn.

MASTER YOUR FUEL SYSTEMS—OR STAY FAT AND TIRED

Obese bodies are unnatural—we all know that.

But so are shredded bodybuilder ones.

At first glance, an obese person and a jacked bodybuilder couldn't seem more different. One is carrying around hundreds of extra pounds, struggling to move with ease. The other is sculpted like a Greek statue, muscles popping in all directions.

But would you find either in nature?

Nature didn't design us to be massive—whether in fat or muscle. *The human body is built for efficiency.* In the wild, excess weight—whether from stored fat or overgrown muscles—was a liability. The bigger you were, the more energy you needed to survive. And in an environment where food wasn't guaranteed, carrying around unnecessary bulk could mean the difference between life and death.

So why do we see so many people at these extremes today? Because we've lost touch with how the body is supposed to work. Both obesity and extreme muscle mass are symptoms of the same problem: a total misunderstanding of the body's fuel system.

Obese people are stuck in constant glucose-burning mode, shoveling in sugar and refined carbs, spiking their insulin, and locking their fat stores away like an untouchable bank vault. Their bodies never access fat for fuel because insulin won't let them.

Bodybuilders, on the other hand, force-feed themselves carbs to fuel insane muscle growth, overloading their systems with glucose. Sure, they might look like peak physical specimens, but their bodies are metabolically fragile, constantly needing to be fed to maintain that artificial mass.

Neither is optimal. Neither is what nature intended. And neither can be sustained long-term without serious consequences. The key to breaking out of this modern mess is understanding your body's two fuel systems—glucose and fat—and learning how to use them the way nature intended.

In this chapter, we're diving into how the body creates and uses energy, why ketosis is the superior fuel source, and how modern diets have completely screwed up our metabolic health. When you grasp how your body is meant to function, you'll never look at food—or fitness—the same way again.

YOUR BODY HAS TWO FUEL SYSTEMS

Your body is a finely tuned engine, but most people have no idea how to fuel it properly. At its core, your body runs on two primary energy systems: glucose metabolism and fatty acid metabolism, also known as ketosis.

Understanding how these two fuel sources work—and when to use them—is the key to unlocking better energy, fat loss, and long-term health.

Let's briefly explain both.

GLUCOSE METABOLISM: THE DEFAULT FUEL

Most people operate almost exclusively on glucose. Every time you eat carbohydrates—bread, pasta, rice, fruit—your body converts them into glucose (sugar) for energy.

Now, glucose *is* important. Certain cells, like your red blood cells, require small amounts of it to function properly. Your body, however, is highly intelligent. It doesn't *need* you to eat carbs to get glucose. It's fully capable of making its own through a process called gluconeogenesis, where the liver converts amino acids from protein into glucose. I'll break that process down more later.

The truth is that your body only needs about *one teaspoon of sugar* circulating in your bloodstream at any given time. For comparison, one cup of basmati rice breaks down into about eleven teaspoons of sugar.

So what happens when you overload your system with more sugar than it needs? Your body treats it like a toxin. High blood sugar triggers insulin release, which works overtime to store the excess as fat (more on insulin soon). Over time, constantly flooding your system with sugar leads to insulin resistance, metabolic dysfunction, and a whole host of modern diseases—obesity, diabetes, heart disease, and even Alzheimer's (now being called "type 3 diabetes").

KETOSIS: THE FAT-BURNING MODE YOUR BODY CRAVES

Your body has a second, more efficient fuel source—fat. When you restrict carbohydrates, your insulin levels drop, and your body starts breaking down stored fat for energy, producing ketones in the process. This is ketosis.

Ketones are a cleaner, more stable energy source than glucose. They provide steady fuel without the energy crashes that come with sugar. But most people never tap into this system because they're constantly eating carbs, keeping insulin levels high, and blocking their body from burning fat.

You may not know this, but your body is designed to enter ketosis.

Historically, humans didn't have 24/7 access to food, let alone sugar. They ate when they could, often going extended periods without food. Their bodies adapted by running on fat.

Your DNA still expects you to operate this way.

Unfortunately, modern diets keep us stuck in glucose-burning mode. Think about it—humans in Boston now eat bananas in February. That's not how nature is supposed to work. We're not meant to have sugar on demand, year-round. Our bodies were built for cyclical eating, alternating between feasting and fasting.

This sugar-driven cycle is why metabolic diseases are skyrocketing. Type 2 diabetes is at epidemic levels, and Alzheimer's is linked to insulin resistance in the brain. PCOS? That's diabetes of the ovaries. Even heart disease is now being traced back to sugar and insulin resistance, not dietary fat (*fuck you, Ancel Keys!*).

Take a look at people with heart disease. Almost all of them are insulin resistant, prediabetic, or carrying excess visceral fat—the dangerous fat that suffocates organs, clogs arteries, and leads to heart attacks. So mastering ketosis isn't just about fat loss, it's about breaking free from this toxic cycle. It's about lowering insulin, burning fat efficiently, and giving your body the metabolic flexibility to function how it was designed to.

The Science of Ketones (A.K.A. Your Body's Superpower)

Ketones are what your body makes when it's burning fat for fuel, and there's more to them than just providing energy. They're like a secret weapon for healing, longevity, and straight-up feeling amazing. It's the key to getting sexy, girlfriend! And not just because you'll lose weight. Science has been all over this for years, and the benefits keep stacking up. Here are three of the most powerful ways ketones work their magic:

1. **Your brain's favorite fuel:** If your brain could talk, it would be shouting, "Feed me ketones!" Unlike glucose, which can cause

crashes and brain fog, ketones provide a steady, clean-burning energy source that keeps your mind clear and focused. That's why ketogenic diets have been used to treat epilepsy since the 1920s—and why researchers are now studying ketones as a therapeutic tool for Alzheimer's, Parkinson's, and other neurodegenerative conditions. Ketones reduce inflammation and oxidative stress in the brain, helping protect against cognitive decline and keeping your neurons firing like they should.

2. **Supercharged endurance and recovery:** The US military taps into the performance-boosting power of ketones. Studies show that ketones help the body use oxygen more efficiently, which means enhanced endurance, better breath control, and faster recovery. That's right—ketones make your body use oxygen more efficiently. It's like your cells go into beast mode, delivering top-tier performance and recovery. Your mitochondria (the little engines inside your cells) run smoother and longer on ketones, allowing you to push harder in workouts, recover faster afterward, and maintain stamina even under extreme physical stress.

3. **Your Body's Cleanup Crew:** Ketones aren't just fuel; they're also regenerative. When ketone levels rise, they trigger autophagy, the body's natural process of cleaning out damaged cells and replacing them with new ones. Think of it as a built-in detox and repair system. On top of that, ketones support tissue healing, reduce inflammation, and improve vascular function, helping keep your heart and arteries in top shape. It's like giving your body an internal tune-up—one that boosts longevity, resilience, and overall vitality.

That's the power of ketones—they don't just fuel your body, they *upgrade* it. But in order to tap into that superpower, you have to stop running on sugar and start managing the real villain behind your cravings, crashes, and chronic fatigue: insulin.

INSULIN: THE ULTIMATE FAT-STORING HORMONE

If you want to understand why most women struggle to burn fat and stay in ketosis, you need to understand *insulin*.

Insulin is a hormone designed to regulate blood sugar and store fat, which is great in small, controlled amounts. But most people live in a *constant state of insulin overload*, thanks to modern high-carb diets.

Every time you eat carbohydrates—whether it's a piece of bread or a bowl of rice—your blood sugar spikes. In response, your pancreas releases insulin to shuttle that sugar into your cells for energy.

Now this part is important: *when insulin is present, your body can't burn fat.*

Insulin *locks your fat stores down like a vault*, forcing your body to rely solely on sugar for fuel. And in today's world, where women are eating carbs all day, every day, *insulin never drops.* This means fat-burning is permanently shut off, and the result is the current metabolic shitshow we see today.

Since high blood sugar is toxic, your body does everything it can to clear it out fast. Insulin plays the role of the cleanup crew, sweeping up excess sugar from your bloodstream. But when sugar floods your system too often, insulin gets stuck in overdrive, locking your body in a vicious cycle of sugar crashes, cravings, and fat storage.

Here's how it works:

1. You eat a high-carb meal, and your blood sugar spikes.
2. Your body releases a surge of insulin, which moves sugar into your cells and converts the excess into fat.
3. Your blood sugar crashes, leaving you tired, hungry, and craving more sugar.
4. You eat again, and the cycle repeats.

Over time, this constant cycle leads to insulin resistance, where your cells stop responding to insulin, forcing your body to pump out even more. Eventually, the system breaks down, leading to pre-diabetes, diabetes, and metabolic dysfunction.

This is why modern high-carb diets are keeping people fat and sick. When you eat carbs all the time, insulin never drops, fat never gets burned, and your body becomes a storage unit instead of a furnace.

And that brings us to one of the most overlooked truths about the human body: *fat is the diamond of the body.*

Your body treats fat like treasure—and for good reason. Fat is the most energy-dense, long-lasting fuel source we have. It's not just excess weight sitting on your hips or belly; it's a biological investment. Think of your body like a savings account. Carbs are the loose change—easy come, easy go. Fat is the diamond—valuable, efficient, and stored away for when things get tough.

As you know, our biology is wired for famine. We evolved to survive long periods without food, and fat was the ticket. It kept us alive through harsh winters, failed hunts, and seasons of scarcity. That's why your body protects fat stores so fiercely. It doesn't see fat as a burden; it sees it as insurance. Something to guard, preserve, and only tap into when absolutely necessary.

And fat isn't just fuel; it's essential. We need fat to build hormones, insulate nerves, support the immune system, and feed the brain. Cholesterol, often demonized in modern health narratives, is actually a building block for sex hormones and cellular repair—and it's made from fat. Your big, beautiful brain is nearly 60 percent fat. Put simply, without fat, you can't think clearly, regulate your hormones, or function at your best.

In today's world of constant snacking, high-carb meals, and never-ending sugar hits, we never give our bodies a chance to cash in on our diamonds. Insulin stays elevated, and as long as insulin is high, your body won't touch its fat stores. Instead, it keeps packing them away, convinced that famine is coming—even though the chances of that are pretty much fucking zilch.

That's the metabolic trap. You're storing diamonds like your life depends on it, but you're never cashing them in. Instead, you stay stuck—always hungry, always tired, and always storing more than you're using.

The only way to break free is to bring insulin down, stop relying on sugar, and give your body permission to do what it was built to do: burn fat.

CARBS ARE NOT ESSENTIAL

This tends to piss a lot of normies off, but *carbohydrates are not required for survival.* That's not an opinion—it's a scientific fact. Unlike protein and fat, which are essential for life, there is no biological requirement for dietary carbohydrates.

Think about it: How did people survive for 150,000 years before agriculture? There were no strawberries in January. No quinoa. No kale. Most carbohydrate-rich plants didn't exist until we started selectively breeding them about ten thousand years ago. So what the hell did we eat? We ate meat, fish, and fat, and we thrived. Our bodies adapted perfectly, using fat and protein as fuel, just as nature intended.

Carbs aren't necessary—they're just a convenient source of quick energy. But in today's world, where they're available 24/7, they've become a metabolic disaster. Sure, our ancestors occasionally ate seasonal fruit or honey, but that was rare. Today, we're eating like it's harvest season every single day of the year. That's not natural.

People on the internet lose their little minds when they hear me say that carbs aren't essential. They'll argue, "But the body needs glucose!"—as if that automatically makes dietary carbohydrates necessary.

It does not, thanks to the process I mentioned earlier called gluconeogenesis. Let's get into it.

Around 30 percent of the protein you eat goes toward building and repairing tissues—muscles, bones, skin, and organs. The rest can be converted into glucose through gluconeogenesis, providing a slow, steady supply of energy. So while glucose is important, dietary carbohydrates are not. Your body is fully capable of producing all the glucose it needs without a single slice of bread, a spoonful of rice, or a piece of fruit.

It's also worth noting that gluconeogenesis is nothing like eating sugar or carbs, which dump glucose into your bloodstream all at once, triggering a massive insulin spike. Instead, glucose from protein is regulated and controlled, keeping blood sugar stable. Think about the difference between chewing a piece of meat and chewing a teaspoon of rice. Rice practically melts in your mouth and is quickly dissolved by stomach acid, flooding your bloodstream with sugar almost instantly. This leads to a sharp spike in blood sugar levels. Meat, on the other hand, takes longer to digest, creating a steady, gentle rise in glucose that sustains your energy throughout the day.

Modern diets and gym culture have further distorted our relationship with carbs. Gym bros who swear by carb-loading argue that they need it for energy, but everything they think they're getting from carbs can also be achieved through a diet of meat and fat. Countless athletes, competitors, and bodybuilders have proven that a carnivore diet supports intense physical activity without the need for carbs.

Still not convinced? Just look at Tom—he's a type 1 diabetic who wears a continuous glucose monitor 24/7. When he eats nothing but meat, his blood sugar still rises. How could that be? *Gluconeogenesis, baby*. His body is converting protein into the exact amount of glucose it needs, no carbs required. This isn't a theory—it's hard data, tracked in real time. His glucose doesn't spike like it would from eating a bowl of rice, but there's a slow, steady increase, proving exactly what I've been saying all along: carbs are not fucking essential.

KETO GONE WRONG: MISTAKES TO AVOID

A lot of women jump into keto thinking it's a magic bullet. They cut carbs, load up on fat, and expect the weight to melt off. And at first, it might. They lose some weight, feel great, and think they've cracked the code—until they plateau. Or worse, they start gaining back the weight. Suddenly, they're blaming keto.

"Keto stopped working for me."

"I must be broken."

No, you're not broken—you just don't understand how your body's fuel system works.

The biggest mistake I see women make when they try keto is not understanding *insulin*—the ultimate fat-storing hormone, as you now know. It doesn't matter how many carbs you cut if you're still triggering an insulin response in ways you don't realize. And when insulin is high, your fat is *locked away*, unavailable for fuel.

There are two big reasons why women struggle with keto: they never truly get into ketosis, or they damage their metabolism by doing keto the wrong way.

Let's break it down and identify the four most common mistakes.

MISTAKE #1: EATING TOO MUCH FAT INSTEAD OF BURNING YOUR OWN

Women hear that ketones are made from fat, so they think, *If I eat more fat, I'll make more ketones.* But sorry, that's not how it works. Your body is incredibly efficient. If it has an easy source of dietary fat, it'll burn that *before* it ever taps into your stored fat. That's why you see people eating 200 grams of fat a day on keto and still not losing weight. They're burning the butter they're eating, not the fat on their body.

We are designed this way for a reason. Remember, fat is the diamond of the body. It's precious. Your body doesn't want to tap into it unless it absolutely has to. In nature, we'd store up fat during the abundant seasons and burn it off in times of scarcity. But today, as pointed out earlier, there's no scarcity. We just keep eating and keep storing. If you want to tap into your stored fat, you have to give your body a reason to use it.

This is why fasting works so well: it forces your body to rely on its own fat stores instead of just burning the fat you eat.

MISTAKE #2: NOT UNDERSTANDING HOW DIETARY FAT CAUSES OVERPRODUCTION OF INSULIN

Some women think keto means they can eat as much fatty food as they want. They pile on butter, drown everything in heavy cream, and eat bacon by the pound, thinking they're golden. But then they're shocked when they don't get into ketosis—or worse, they start gaining weight. So what's happening?

Answer: insulin doesn't just spike from carbs, it also rises in response to excess fat if you're eating it alongside protein.

Say you're eating a big, juicy ribeye. Protein naturally breaks down into glucose *slowly* through that process you learned about earlier called gluconeogenesis. But when you add a ton of fat—think butter, heavy cream, or excessive cheese—it slows everything down even more. Your body has to work harder to process it, excreting more insulin, keeping you loaded with the master fat-storing hormone.

And as long as insulin is up, *you're not burning fat.*

This is why so many women think they're in ketosis when they're not. They might even use those urine ketone strips, which are useless after the first couple of weeks. If you're serious about knowing whether you're in ketosis, you need to test your blood ketone levels. Otherwise, you're flying blind.

MISTAKE #3: HIGH-FAT, LOW-PROTEIN KETO (A RECIPE FOR METABOLIC SLOWDOWN)

Some women take keto to the extreme and try to "hack" the system by cutting back on protein. They fear protein will spike their blood sugar, so they eat tiny portions of meat and drown everything in butter and MCT oil.

But your body absolutely needs protein.

Protein isn't just another macronutrient—it's the foundation of your body. Every cell, every muscle, every organ relies on protein for repair and function. When you limit protein, like the high-fat, low-protein "keto diet" advises, you don't eat enough and your body burns through its glycogen stores first. Then, once those are gone, it starts *breaking down muscle* to make the glucose it needs.

This is where the real damage happens. Your body realizes it's in trouble—it's eating itself alive. So it slams the brakes on your metabolism. Your thyroid slows down, your energy plummets, and your body starts clinging to every calorie like it's the last one it'll ever see. This is why so many women who do keto incorrectly feel sluggish and struggle to lose weight long-term.

In my experience, most women do not eat enough protein to begin with, so limiting your protein is the last thing you should do.

MISTAKE #4: CHASING HIGH KETONE NUMBERS INSTEAD OF FAT LOSS

Some women become obsessed with their ketone levels, trying to get them as high as possible by chugging MCT oil or taking exogenous ketones. And sure, you can artificially boost your ketones this way, but why? The whole point of keto is to burn *your own fat*, not just make ketones for the sake of seeing a high number on a test strip.

Your body naturally makes ketones from saturated fat, which comes from animal foods, not from plant oils. While coconut oil and palm oil are exceptions because they contain saturated fat, most plant oils—like olive oil—don't directly contribute to ketone production. So if you're relying on processed oils instead of prioritizing natural animal fats, you're missing the point.

The bottom line? Keto isn't broken—you're just *doing it wrong*. Instead of trying to "hack" your metabolism with shortcuts, you need to work with nature, not against it:

- Burn your own fat first before loading up on dietary fat.
- Be mindful of insulin. It's not just about carbs; fat and protein play a role too.
- Eat enough protein so your body doesn't eat its own muscle.
- Don't use synthetic ketones; use your own.

The best biohack isn't a supplement, a fancy oil, or some over-priced powder—it's understanding *how your body actually works.*

TOM'S TAKE: THE TRUTH ABOUT
KETOACIDOSIS VS. KETOSIS

Ketoacidosis and ketosis get thrown around like they're the same thing, but they couldn't be more different. So let's clear this up once and for all.

Ketoacidosis is a serious, life-threatening condition that happens *almost exclusively* in type 1 diabetics like me. It occurs when ketone levels skyrocket uncontrollably because there's no insulin to regulate them. Without insulin, the body can't use glucose for energy, so it starts breaking down fat at an extreme rate, flooding the blood with ketones and turning it dangerously acidic. If left untreated, this can lead to organ failure, coma, or death.

Sounds scary, right? It is, but only if you're a type 1 diabetic or in some other rare, extreme metabolic state.

For the rest of you? *Ketoacidosis is not a concern.* Your body has built-in mechanisms to prevent it. The moment your ketone levels start getting too high, insulin is released to bring them back down. Even if you're fasting or in deep ketosis, your pancreas steps in to keep things balanced.

Your body knows exactly what to do.

But for type 1 diabetics like me, it's a different story. Since my body doesn't make insulin, I have to be careful. If I don't manage my insulin properly and my blood sugar skyrockets, my ketones can get out of control. But even then, ketoacidosis doesn't just happen instantly. It takes time—usually *hours to days* of mismanagement. There are even undiagnosed type 1 diabetics who walk around in ketoacidosis for months before realizing something's wrong. That's how resilient the body is, even under extreme conditions.

So if you're not type 1 diabetic, you do not need to worry about keto-acidosis. Ketosis is a natural, safe, and preferred metabolic state for humans. Stop letting fear-mongering about ketoacidosis keep you from tapping into the metabolic benefits of ketosis.

MITOCHONDRIA: YOUR BODY'S BUILT-IN POWER PLANTS

Your body is a high-performance machine, and like any machine, its energy production matters. That's where our mitochondria come in. These tiny powerhouses inside your cells are responsible for turning fuel into energy—and how efficiently they do that depends on what kind of fuel you're giving them.

Mitochondria play many roles, so you'll see them pop up in the next few chapters. In this chapter, we'll look at how these cellular engines interact with our modern food systems—and what that means for energy, metabolism, and long-term health. In Chapter 5, we'll explore how mitochondria respond to the sun. And in Chapter 6, we'll dive into their relationship with circadian rhythms.

Before we dig into how our food choices affect mitochondrial function, let's take a quick refresher on these little powerhouses. Mitochondria take the food you eat and convert it into ATP (adenosine triphosphate)—the energy currency that powers everything from your heartbeat to your brain function. They can run on glucose (from carbs) or fat (which produces ketones), but most people never give their mitochondria a break from running on glucose.

And here's a little secret: your mitochondria prefer fat as fuel.

Burning fat and ketones makes your mitochondria far more efficient. Instead of generating a ton of metabolic waste (which happens with glucose), ketones burn cleaner, cooler, and produce more energy with less oxidative stress. It's like switching from low-grade fuel to premium—everything just runs better.

I mentioned earlier that certain cells in your body (like red blood cells) need glucose. One of the reasons is because these cells don't have mitochondria, so they *must* use glucose. But for pretty much everything else, your body sees ketones as the superior fuel. Even your brain prefers ketones over glucose.

This brings me to the question: Why prioritize fat as a fuel source? It's not just about weight loss or hopping on the latest diet trend; it's about tapping into the most metabolically efficient and restorative fuel system your body has.

When you burn fat, your mitochondria produce ketones—and when they're running on ketones instead of glucose, the difference is astonishing. For instance, 100 grams of beta-hydroxybutyrate (one of the primary ketones) can yield 10.5 kg of ATP, while 100 grams of glucose yields 8.7 kg of ATP. That means more ATP is produced per molecule of oxygen, and far less oxidative stress is created in the process. In other words, ketones offer a cleaner, cooler, and quieter energy.

Oxidative stress is one of the root causes of cellular aging and chronic disease. So when your mitochondria run on fat, they generate energy without the metabolic smoke and friction that comes with glucose. That translates to better cellular performance across the board—your muscles recover faster, your brain stays sharper, and your entire system operates with greater resilience and longevity.

By shifting your body into fat-burning mode, you're not just optimizing your energy and getting sexy in the process—you're unlocking your biology's original design for health, repair, and endurance.

THE WARBURG EFFECT: HOW GLUCOSE OVERLOAD FUELS CANCER

If optimizing your mitochondria with fat didn't already convince you to ditch carbs, maybe this will: cancer cells *love* sugar. They're addicted to it. Feed them glucose and they thrive. Cut off their supply and they struggle. This isn't some fringe theory—it's a phenomenon first discovered in the 1920s by Nobel Prize-winning scientist Dr. Otto Warburg.

Warburg found that cancer cells don't play by the same metabolic rules as healthy cells. Instead of using oxygen-efficient mitochondria to produce energy, they switch to fermentation—even when oxygen is available. This is called the Warburg Effect, and it's one of the hallmarks of cancer metabolism.

Here's what that means in simple terms:

- Healthy cells use the Krebs cycle to generate energy—clean, efficient, oxygen-based.
- Cancer cells bypass this system and ferment glucose into lactic acid, a chaotic and inefficient process that creates more metabolic waste.
- This fermentation allows them to survive in damaged, inflamed, oxygen-deprived environments—conditions that sugar consumption helps create.

Cancer cells are glucose junkies. Warburg's research suggests that too much glucose in the system can create the perfect breeding ground for them to thrive. So if you're flooding your body with sugar, you're rolling out the red carpet for disease.

In Chapter 1, when I said cancer was a choice, this is why.

Since we've already established that your body is a race car, let's take the analogy further. Think of glucose as cheap, low-quality fuel that burns hot, overheating your system, creating oxidative stress, and accelerating damage. Over time, this chronic inflammation can lead to metabolic chaos—including cancer.

Ketones, on the other hand, are premium fuel. As we shared in the last section, they burn cooler and cleaner, reducing oxidative stress and protecting your mitochondria from unnecessary wear and tear.

This is why ketosis has been studied as a potential therapy for cancer—not because it's a magic cure, but because it creates a metabolic environment where healthy cells thrive and cancer cells struggle.

Now, I am not claiming that ketones cure cancer, but I am saying this: the way we fuel our bodies matters—deeply. When you prioritize clean-burning fat over sugar, you create conditions that support cellular health and resilience. And in a world where cancer continues to rise, understanding the metabolic roots of disease isn't just helpful, it's essential.

FORGET THE TECH; YOU ARE NATURE

If we traveled back in time just a few hundred years, would you see people carb-loading before a hunt? Strapping glucose monitors to their arms? Tracking macros in an app? Of course not. They didn't need to. They lived in harmony with the rhythms of the earth—fasting when food was scarce, feasting when it was available, and running on fat more often than not.

Unfortunately, we've overcomplicated everything today. Gym culture has people convinced they need massive muscles to be fit. Diet culture has people guzzling MCT oil to "hack" ketosis. Wellness culture has people tracking their glucose like it's the stock market. But none of this is natural.

It's modern-day fuckery.

You don't need a glucose monitor to tell you what happens when you eat a cinnamon roll. You should fucking know by now.

We've become domesticated—trained to rely on external data instead of internal cues. We micromanage our diets like we're feeding lab rats, constantly second-guessing hunger, energy, sleep, and mood, instead of just tuning in. And the more we rely on tech and trackers, the further we drift from the wild intelligence our bodies were born with.

Take continuous glucose monitors (CGMs), for example. People slap them on and obsess over every little spike like it's the full picture. But it's not. CGMs show glucose—not insulin. So if your blood sugar looks fine but your insulin is constantly spiking behind the scenes, that monitor isn't catching the storm—it's just reporting the calm before it. You could be on the fast track to insulin resistance and have no clue.

I've seen this too many times:

"My blood sugar has always been in the 80s—how am I prediabetic?"

"I track everything! Why didn't anyone warn me?"

Because insulin resistance doesn't knock politely. It builds quietly for years—decades even—and then one day, your body taps out. You go from "I'm fine" to "How the hell did this happen?" overnight.

But you don't need a warning label if you're paying attention, girlfriend.

Are you eating sugar and refined carbs every day? Drinking soda, snacking constantly, skipping fat, and chasing every crash with caffeine? If so, you're not in harmony with nature.

At the end of the day, you don't need the gadgets—you need to understand your fuel systems. Burning glucose is fast, hot, and dirty. It gives you quick energy but leaves behind a metabolic mess. Burning fat, on the other hand, is slow, clean, and efficient. It fuels long-lasting energy, protects your mitochondria, and keeps your system cool.

When you eat real food and give your body space between meals, it shifts naturally into fat-burning mode. That's what you're designed to do. That's nature's default.

So no, you don't need more hacks or more tech. You just need to remember what you are. You are nature. Your body already knows the way as long as you're not standing in the way.

YOU WERE DESIGNED TO THRIVE

Everything about our biology was built for efficiency. You weren't meant to be on an energy roller coaster, crashing and craving every few hours. You weren't designed to haul around excess fat that your body refuses to burn. And you sure as hell weren't wired to rely on constant glucose hits just to function.

You were meant to move with nature, not fight against it.

Unfortunately, the modern world has hijacked that design. Now we celebrate extremes—obesity on one end, shredded bodybuilders on the other—both metabolically broken in their own ways. One can't burn fat; the other lives on glucose and stimulants to maintain a body that looks "fit" but runs on fumes. Neither is natural. Neither is sustainable. And neither understands how the body was meant to fuel itself.

Ketosis is the original operating system. It's how our ancestors went days without food and still had the clarity and strength to hunt, think, and lead. It's how the body heals and protects itself—from inflammation, from degeneration, and yes, even from cancer.

When you align with how your body was designed to work, everything gets easier. Mastering your fuel systems isn't some diet trend either. It's returning to the metabolic flexibility your ancestors had. It's about reclaiming the ability to burn fat the way you were built to.

It's how our ancestors stayed raw, radiant, and sexy without trying.

When you master your fuel systems, you get sexy too—just like nature intended.

PRINCIPLE #5

WORSHIP THE SUN

"The sun causes cancer."

"I burn too easily."

"I never leave the house without sunscreen on."

Sound familiar?

These are the stories we've been told for decades—repeated so often that they've calcified into belief. But did you know that low vitamin D levels are directly linked to *increased cancer risk*? That's right. The very thing we've been told to avoid for fear of cancer is actually one of the most powerful tools for preventing it.

Don't believe me? The studies are out there. One massive meta-analysis found that people with the lowest vitamin D levels had a 14 percent higher cancer mortality rate than those with the highest levels.[1] And I'm not just talking about skin cancer. Breast cancer. Colon cancer. Prostate cancer. Multiple myeloma. Across the board, the risk goes up as vitamin D goes down.

So let's ask some obvious questions: Why is it that as sunscreen

---

[1]   Ben Schöttker et al., "Vitamin D and Mortality: Meta-Analysis of Individual Participant Data from a Large Consortium of Cohort Studies from Europe and the United States," *BMJ* 348 (2014): g3656, https://doi.org/10.1136/bmj.g3656.

use has skyrocketed, skin cancer rates have climbed right alongside it? Why do hunter-gatherer tribes who live outside every day—with no sunscreen, no hats, no sunglasses—have some of the lowest cancer rates on the planet? If the sun is so dangerous, how did humans survive for so long without SPF?

The root answer to all of these questions is—you guessed it!—because we've been domesticated away from the sun (and straight-up lied to about it).

The truth is we were designed to worship the sun, not fear it. It sets our circadian rhythm. It charges our mitochondria. It signals our hormones. It boosts our immune function. And yes, the sun helps us make vitamin D, one of the most essential nutrients for human health.

The sun is not a threat.

It's the original life source.

In the modern world, however, we've traded that life source for fluorescent lights, LED screens, and ten-hour stretches indoors. We slather ourselves in chemical sunscreens, avoid natural light, and then wonder why we're anxious, exhausted, insulin-resistant, and inflamed.

Everything you've been taught about the sun is wrong. This chapter is about undoing the damage. It's about unlearning the lies we've been sold about sun exposure, sunscreen, and blue light—and rebuilding a relationship with natural light that supports our biology. You'll learn how melanin works, why vitamin D is so much more than a supplement, and how to sync back up with the light cycles that shaped human evolution.

Because worshiping the sun isn't just a catchy principle—it's how you get sexy, girlfriend!

THE SUN IS A NUTRIENT

We've been taught to treat the sun like a monster—something to block, avoid, and fear. But the sun isn't just light—it's a nutrient.

And I don't mean that in a vague, life-affirming kind of way. In the same way your body needs magnesium, protein, or B12 to function properly, it needs sunlight.

Let's start with what most people *do* know: the sun helps you make vitamin D. When UVB rays hit your skin, they convert cholesterol into vitamin D3, which then gets activated by your liver and kidneys into a hormone that affects everything from calcium absorption to immune regulation. So yes, sunlight is a crucial part of how your body maintains health.

But sunlight is far more than a vitamin D delivery system.

To reduce sunlight to "just vitamin D" is like reducing food to calories. It's missing the bigger picture. When full-spectrum UVB light hits your skin, you're not just making D. You're kicking off a cascade of biological processes that no supplement can replicate. Sunlight is biological information. It tells your body what time it is, what hormones to produce, when to sleep, when to wake, when to burn fat, and when to heal.

Light enters your eyes and hits specialized cells in your retina, signaling the brain's suprachiasmatic nucleus—your master circadian clock. That signal orchestrates hormone release, metabolism, mood, and sleep-wake cycles. Morning sunlight helps suppress melatonin, boost cortisol (in a good way), and elevate serotonin—all of which improve energy, focus, and resilience.

And then there's your mitochondria—those little power plants inside your cells. Red and near-infrared light from the sun penetrates deep into tissues and literally charges your cells, enhancing ATP (energy) production. This is something no supplement can mimic. It's why getting outside often makes you feel more energized and alive.

Even your immune system responds to light. Sunlight helps regulate T cells, reduce inflammation, and strengthen the body's defense against pathogens. Some research even shows that natural light exposure improves wound healing and reduces the severity of autoimmune flares. Sunlight also boosts nitric oxide production, which improves blood flow, supports heart health, and may help regulate blood pressure.

This is why we must worship the sun, girlfriend!

Yet today, we treat sunlight like it's optional. Something nice if you happen to go for a walk. A guilty pleasure if you sit outside too long. But if something is essential to your survival, to your optimal functioning, to your energy, mood, and immune system—it's not a luxury; it's a requirement.

And like any nutrient, when you don't get enough, you suffer. Low energy. Hormonal disruption. Depression. Immune dysfunction. Increased cancer risk. All of it is tied, directly or indirectly, to sunlight deficiency.

It's time to stop treating the sun like a threat and start treating it like the essential nutrient it is.

DOES THE SUN REALLY CAUSE CANCER?

We've all heard that too much sun causes cancer, but is that really true? I question this notion.

I have a lot of fucking questions, actually.

Despite decades of sunscreen marketing and public health campaigns urging sun avoidance, skin cancer rates have continued to rise. In fact, studies have shown a direct correlation between increased sunscreen usage and increased melanoma rates.[2] This is known as the "sunscreen paradox."

If slathering on SPF were truly protecting us, why are more people being diagnosed with skin cancer than ever before?

A 2016 study published in *Dermato-Endocrinology* noted the paradox directly: as sunscreen use increased, so did melanoma incidence. The authors argued that regular sunscreen application blocks UVB

---

2   Sauliha Alli et al., "Understanding the Perceived Relationship Between Sun Exposure and Melanoma in Atlantic Canada: A Consensual Qualitative Study Highlighting a 'Sunscreen Paradox,'" *Cancers* 15, no. 19 (2023): 4726, https://doi.org/10.3390/cancers15194726.

rays, which are required for vitamin D synthesis, while allowing deeper-penetrating UVA rays through—the exact ones more strongly associated with DNA damage and melanoma.[3]

If sunscreen is marketed as protection, could it be contributing to the problem? And isn't it strange that skin cancer rates are directly connected to low vitamin D? Could it be that those who avoid the sun the most are the ones getting cancer?

A meta-analysis published in *PLOS ONE* (2017) found that individuals with higher vitamin D levels had significantly lower cancer mortality rates across the board.[4] Vitamin D isn't just a bonus nutrient; it's a hormonal regulator that affects everything from immune function to gene expression. With low vitamin D levels consistently linked to higher rates of cancer mortality—not just skin cancer, but also breast, colon, prostate, and multiple myeloma—could it be that a deficiency in this critical nutrient is a larger issue than we've realized?

So why, instead of addressing the root issue—sunlight deficiency—are we doubling down on the fear of the sun?

Modern life has made us solar-phobic. Could our indoor, screen-dominated lifestyles be contributing to the rise in chronic illness? Could the avoidance of natural sunlight be playing a role in the silent epidemic of vitamin D deficiency?

These are questions worth asking. We've been sold the idea that the sun is the problem, when perhaps, it might be the missing ingredient.

WE'VE BEEN DOMESTICATED AWAY FROM THE SUN

If you think you can't handle the sun, it's not because your body is broken—it's because you've been domesticated away from it.

---

3   S.L McDonnell et al., "Serum 25-Hydroxyvitamin D Concentrations ≥40 ng/ml Are Associated with >65% Lower Cancer Risk: Pooled Analysis of Randomized Trial and Prospective Cohort Study," *PLOS ONE* 11, no. 4 (2016): e0152441, https://doi.org/10.1371/journal.pone.0152441.

4   Martin Gaksch et al., "Vitamin D and Mortality: Individual Participant Data Meta-Analysis of Standardized 25-hydroxyvitamin D in 26916 Individuals from a European Consortium," *PLOS ONE* 12, no. 2 (2017): e0170791, https://doi.org/10.1371/journal.pone.0170791.

Most people today live under artificial lights, behind glass, under roofs, in climate-controlled spaces. They go from car to office to home without ever really experiencing natural light. And when they do finally step outside, their skin panics. No solar resilience. No adaptation. Of course they burn—they've given their body zero training.

It's like tossing a city-raised kid into the wilderness and expecting them to thrive. They're not weak. They're just unprepared.

Your skin was built to handle the sun, but like anything in nature, it needs time and consistency to adapt. You don't go from nothing to full-on sun worship overnight. Just like strength training, you build your tolerance gradually. Early morning sun, short bursts of midday exposure, finding shade when you need it—that's how you train your skin to do what it was designed to do.

In case you don't know how your skin works, when UV light hits it, the light triggers the production of melanin, a natural antioxidant and protective mechanism. Melanin doesn't just give your skin color, it protects you from the sun by building resilience. It's your body's way of adapting to the environment, and a tan is simply a deeper biological adaptation. This adaptation isn't cosmetic; it's functional. It allows your skin to handle more sunlight without burning. Tanning is your body's way of becoming stronger and more capable of absorbing light. But when you avoid sunlight and never develop this adaptation, your skin stays weak and fragile, leaving you more prone to burning.

Another form of domestication is the skin type chart. Sheesh. You don't have a "skin type." You simply have skin. And that skin is either adapted to handle sunlight, or it's not. If it's not, that's your fault, not your genetics. Your red hair, your fair skin, your tendency to burn—none of that excludes you from the laws of biology. Our ancestors lived outside in the sun! You are not special. Every cell in your body is a photoreceptor—regardless of your skin color. That means your body is literally wired to interact with sunlight.

Your mitochondria rely on light to function at their best. This isn't some fringe wellness idea—this is basic human physiology. Your body is solar-powered. It was designed to move with the sun, not hide from it.

And nature doesn't care about your excuses, girlfriend. You can argue all day that you "don't tan" or that you "need sunscreen," but that doesn't change the fact that your biology expects sunlight. If you're not giving it what it needs, you're not going to function well. Period.

This conditioning extends to your eyes too.

If you step outside and immediately squint or feel blinded by the light, that's not just sensitivity—it's a sign you've weakened your natural defenses. Again, you've been domesticated. Your eyes are supposed to adjust. They're equipped with built-in mechanisms to regulate light exposure. But if you've been wearing sunglasses every time you leave the house, you've trained your vision to become light-intolerant.

So how do you undo the damage? How do you rewild yourself back to your natural relationship with the sun?

- Build your solar resiliency. Start with small doses of sun. Let your skin gradually adapt. You can't tan in one day—you need consistency over time.
- Stop relying on sunscreen. Let your skin remember how to protect itself. That's its job.
- Lose the sunglasses. Let your eyes relearn how to handle natural light. Give them the signal they've been missing.

You don't need protection from the sun. You need to reclaim your relationship with it.

THINK OF THE SUN AS YOUR CHARGER

We obsess over charging our devices—our phones, laptops, tablets— plugging them in religiously to keep them running. But when was the last time you thought about charging *yourself*?

Think of the sun as your charger. It's been charging life on this planet since the beginning of time. Every living thing—plants, animals, humans—is wired to thrive under its energy.

When you step outside, you're not just soaking up some rays and getting a tan. You're plugging into your original power source. The sun doesn't just give you vitamin D—it sends electromagnetic signals that program your body at the cellular level. It's literally telling your mitochondria to do their job. The sun charges you with energy, repairs your DNA, cools down the oxidative stress your cells create just from living, and programs your hormones like melatonin and insulin to keep you running like the finely tuned machine you were designed to be.

You can't charge yourself by sitting inside or hiding behind sunglasses all day. The glass in your windows blocks most of the beneficial wavelengths, and the artificial lights in your office don't even come close to mimicking the sun's spectrum. That's like trying to charge your phone with a knockoff charger—it's not going to work, and it might even do more harm than good. You need the real deal. You need direct sunlight on your skin and through your eyes.

And just like your phone's battery will eventually degrade if you don't charge it properly, your body will too. When you skip your daily dose of sunlight, you're basically running on empty. Over time, this lack of proper "charging" leads to fatigue, poor sleep, hormonal imbalances, and a whole host of metabolic issues.

And no amount of supplements, coffee, or fancy gadgets will ever fix that.

So start thinking of the sun as your personal charger. Get outside during the day, even if it's cloudy. The sun's energy penetrates through clouds and still does its thing.

THE BLUE LIGHT PROBLEM: WHY YOUR BODY IS SO CONFUSED

Humans were designed to interact with natural light. The sun follows a perfect rhythm—rising with warm reds, oranges, and golds, peaking at noon with the highest concentration of blue light, then fading back into deep reds and purples as it sets. This cycle is what programs our biology. It tells our body when to wake up, when to be alert, when to eat, and when to wind down for sleep.

But modern life has hijacked this system.

Instead of following the sun, we wake up to phone screens blasting artificial blue light, sit in front of computers all day under fluorescent bulbs, and then doom-scroll on our phones until we finally shut our eyes. We've replaced the sun's balanced spectrum with constant synthetic blue light, and our bodies are completely lost.

We're biologically confused—perpetually stuck in a "solar noon" state from the moment we wake up until the second we fall asleep. And that confusion has serious consequences.

One of which is dopamine toxicity.

DOPAMINE: THE OTHER BLUE LIGHT DRUG

Being outside in natural sunlight boosts dopamine, which is why stepping into a bright, sunny day feels instantly good. Don't you love looking outside and seeing a blue sky? Don't you love it even more when you sit outside with the sun's rays hitting your face? That's nature rewarding you—encouraging you to get outside and be active.

Unfortunately, blue light has fucked this all up because it hijacks our brain.

Every time you stare at a screen, you're giving yourself a fake dopamine hit. And don't get me started on social media. That's an even bigger dopamine rush. Likes, comments, notifications—they're all designed to keep you coming back for more. And when you flood your system with constant dopamine, congratulations, now you have dopamine toxicity. That's when things really start to go sideways.

Dopamine toxicity isn't just about feeling overstimulated; it's a rewiring of the brain's reward system. Your baseline for pleasure gets so high that regular life starts to feel boring, flat, even unbearable. You need more and more stimulation just to feel *normal*. Meanwhile, your focus tanks, motivation drops, and the things that used to bring you joy—sex, connection, nature—barely register.

Now you get irritable, restless, and aggressive. Your sex hormones get out of whack. Your nervous system gets overloaded. Some studies even suggest that excess dopamine is linked to bipolar disorder and other mental health issues.

That's us fucking with nature again.

This is also why kids lose their minds when you take away their screens. It's not just "kids being kids"; they're going through withdrawal. That tablet has been feeding their dopamine all day long, and when you rip it away, they freak the fuck out. Just like an addict losing access to their fix.

HIJACKED BY FREQUENCY: THE INVISIBLE ASSAULT OF EMFS

If sunlight is your body's operating system, EMFs are the malware.

In this chapter, I've talked about how your body was designed to interact with natural light—how the sun calibrates your hormones, your sleep, and your energy. But that entire system is being hijacked by something you can't see, can't hear, and can't touch: electromagnetic fields.

Wi-Fi, Bluetooth, cell towers, smart devices, your phone, your laptop—even your electric car—all emit invisible radiation that pulses through your environment 24/7. This isn't woo-woo science. Your body is electrical. Every heartbeat, every nerve signal, every thought depends on finely tuned electric currents. And those currents are being disrupted.

You were designed to sync with the earth's gentle magnetic field and the infrared spectrum of the sun—not to marinate in an artificial web of high-frequency signals. But that's exactly what we've done. We've traded the sun and soil for routers and radiation.

And our bodies are paying the price.

IF YOU COULD SEE IT, YOU'D FREAK THE FUCK OUT

If EMFs were visible, your world would look like a war zone. Pulsing waves shooting from your phone, beaming from your router, bouncing off power lines. You'd see your body constantly bombarded by chaotic frequencies—every organ, every cell, every system under pressure. But because it's invisible, we don't even realize what is happening.

Allow me to enlighten you.

Your nervous system starts glitching, leading to stress, poor sleep, and dysregulation. Your immune system gets overwhelmed or worn out. Your hormones shift out of balance—testosterone drops, melatonin tanks, insulin function derails. And your cells become inflamed, confused, and exhausted from trying to adapt to an unnatural environment.

Because the effects are slow, no one connects the dots. Like low arsenic poisoning over time, the symptoms sneak in—fatigue, anxiety, brain fog—and we just chalk it up to stress or age. But after a while, the damage adds up.

So what can we do?

Unfortunately, you can't escape EMFs completely—not unless you're living off-grid in a remote cabin with zero signal and no neighbors for fifty miles. But that doesn't mean you're powerless. Your biology is incredibly resilient, as long as you give it the right inputs.

Here's how to start defending your system and reclaiming your natural frequency:

- **Get back into nature.** Your body speaks the language of sunlight and Earth's magnetic field. Every time you walk barefoot on grass, dirt, or sand, you reconnect with the grounding energy that calms your nervous system and lowers inflammation. Morning sunlight in your eyes resets your circadian rhythm (more on that in the next chapter). Red light and raw earth are the original antianxiety medicine; your body knows exactly what to do with them.
- **Control what you can.** Turn off Wi-Fi at night—your body does

most of its repair work during sleep, and it won't run optimally if it's being bombarded by EMFs all night. Keep your phone out of your bedroom and in airplane mode when possible. Don't put your phone in your bra or pocket. Stop wearing Bluetooth earbuds all day; they basically microwave your brain. You can't remove all the noise, but do your best to mitigate what you can.

- **Support your system.** EMFs are just one piece of the modern stress pile. Your best defense is resilience, which comes from aligning your habits with nature. Eat real food, sleep when it's dark, move your body, and get sunlight in your eyes every morning. These primal inputs tune your body's systems so they can handle more of what the modern world throws at you.

None of us can be perfect. But we can be aware. And that awareness is your first line of defense in a world that's quietly, constantly messing with your biology.

GET SEXY IN THE SUN

It is time to burn the old beliefs, ladies. You know the ones: the warnings you've heard your whole life. The myths about the sun being dangerous. The conditioning that made you think your skin was too sensitive, that sunscreen was survival, that staying inside was somehow safer.

None of it was rooted in truth. It was rooted in fear—and fear is a shitty foundation for health.

You weren't made to hide from nature; you were made to work with it. The sun was your original charger, your circadian rhythm setter, your hormonal regulator. It was never the threat. It was the missing piece.

When you stop hiding from the sun and start rebuilding your relationship with it, your biology responds. Your skin adapts. Your mood lifts. Your energy comes back. This is more than getting outside more. It's about peeling off the layers of domestication and getting back to the raw truth of how your body works. Because that's what this whole thing is about—every principle, every shift. So if you're serious about health, vitality, and yes, becoming sexy from the inside out, embrace the very life force your body depends on.

And since the sun sets the rhythm for everything in your body, I'm not done with it just yet. Up next: circadian hormones, light timing, and how to finally get in sync with your biology.

PRINCIPLE #6

OBEY YOUR CIRCADIAN CLOCK

It's the middle of the night. While you're sleeping (dreaming of sweet nothings), your body is busy following its circadian clock, the internal rhythm designed to keep everything running on time. At around 2:00 a.m., cortisol is released, priming your blood sugar to get you ready for the day. As the sun hits the horizon, your body shuts off melatonin, signaling that it's time to wake up.

That's how it's supposed to go, anyway. But when most women wake up these days, they step into the chaos of modern life, and just fuck it all up.

Let's explore what a typical modern woman's day looks like, shall we?

It's 5:00 a.m. You stumble out of bed groggy, already stressing over the day, and pour yourself a giant cup of coffee. You think this cup of joe is waking you up, but that caffeine only triggers more cortisol (your stress hormone), which jacks up your blood sugar again.

So now your insulin's out, confused, and asking, *What the fuck is happening?* You haven't even eaten, but your body is reacting like you are being chased by a lion. Insulin is trying to manage the chaos, but it is struggling. You grab breakfast—maybe some bullshit avocado toast or overnight oats—and scroll through your phone while eating. Good job. You've got coffee, sugar, and synthetic light working together to blow up your nervous system, causing a tidal wave of insulin before you've even left the house.

Then, instead of moving your body like it's designed to, you plant your ass in the car for an hour-long commute to work. You're pissed off at traffic, flipping people off, and stressing about your shitty job. By the time you roll into the office to sit at your desk, you've spent the entire morning pumping insulin without burning off a single drop of glucose.

Congrats, you're literally sitting there *getting fatter.*

At the office, you plop down under fluorescent lights in front of a giant blue screen. Your skin hasn't seen the sun at all—except for the two seconds it took you to walk from your car to the building. Your blood sugar stays sky-high because, again, you're not moving.

By lunchtime, you're drained. Your blood sugar tanks, your adrenals are fried, and you're desperate for a pick-me-up. So you head to Panera, scarf down a grilled cheese and a salad, pat yourself on the back for eating veggies, and then grab another coffee because you're dead inside. That meal spikes your blood sugar—*again*—and insulin comes barreling in like a stressed-out mom at Target, juggling a meltdown and a cart full of regrets.

Meanwhile, your mitochondria are working overtime just to keep you alive. They're overheating, creating oxidative stress, and guess what's supposed to cool them down? Ketones, which you aren't producing because you're burning glucose and not fat.

You're literally *rusting* from the inside out.

Let's fast-forward to the gym now. You chug a protein shake—a glorified milkshake that hits your insulin like a damn freight train—and head under bright blue lights to sweat it out with the other clueless gym rats. Your blood sugar crashes because of all the insulin, leaving you starving. You go home, order from Uber Eats because you're too tired to cook, and binge on whatever greasy crap shows up at your door. Now it's 8:00 p.m. You're scrolling on your phone, bathing in more blue light, and wondering why you can't fall asleep.

Well, I'll tell you why, girlfriend: your body thinks it's still daytime because of all the artificial light, so melatonin—your nighttime repair crew—never shows up. You toss and turn, wired and exhausted, waking up the next morning to repeat the same exhausting cycle.

When your system is *this* broken, how the hell are you supposed to feel sexy? How are you going to have a sex drive? Or the energy to live your life? Your body's not interested in thriving when it's busy trying to survive.

Let's contrast this common reality with what it would have been like for you if you were a Native American or a Viking.

In other words, how nature intended us to live.

WHAT NATURE INTENDED

The day begins before the sun fully rises, with a soft wash of dawn spilling across the sky. You wake naturally, your body perfectly attuned to the earth's rhythm. No alarm clock, no jolting buzz—just cortisol gently stirring you from sleep. Resting on animal pelts spread on the ground has kept you grounded through the night, your nervous system synced to the hum of the planet.

At first light, you move your body. You gather water from a stream, check traps, or rekindle the fire. If it's cold, you start a broth with bones and meat from the night before. This first meal isn't a rushed grab-and-go. It's a ritual—a way to fuel your body with the warmth and nourishment it needs for the work ahead. The food is simple, nutrient-dense, and unprocessed: animal fat and protein.

As the sun climbs, it speaks to your body in a language of light. It tells your mitochondria to produce energy, balances your hormones, and begins the slow programming of melatonin for the night to come. Your skin absorbs its rays, your eyes soak in its spectrum. You feel awake, alive, fully charged.

The day is spent in purposeful movement and connection. You walk miles—not because you need to count steps, but because your survival depends on it. If you hunt, you do so with patience, skill, and reverence. If you forage, you read the land like a book passed down through generations. Every movement is functional. Every action matters. There is no "exercise." Your body becomes strong because your life demands it.

If you're not hunting or gathering, your hands are busy with the work of the village—preparing food, fixing tools, weaving fibers into rope or baskets. Children learn by shadowing you, mimicking every move. Elders offer stories and wisdom, holding space for guidance, not retirement.

Meals are shared. When food is plentiful, the whole community eats together—meat, fish, seasonal berries. You sit in a circle, not at a screen. You talk. You laugh. You rest. Eating is not just sustenance, it's celebration.

As the sun dips, the pace slows. You return home with game or goods, settling in for the evening. There's no artificial light, just a crackling fire. The sky turns to ink and fills with stars—your original calendar, your map, your reminder that you belong to something vast. Your body, already winding down, begins its descent into sleep. Melatonin rises. There's no fight against it. You lie down close to others, sharing warmth and space. Your body, recharged by sun and effort, slips easily into deep, regenerative rest.

In summer, the days stretch and food is abundant. In winter, the nights come early, and fasting happens naturally. You don't resist the seasons; you move with them. This is what nature intended.

How dreamy would that be?

Nature gave us a blueprint, and we're out here coloring outside the lines with a Sharpie. Now, obviously we live in a modern world and living like our ancestors is not 100 percent possible. But we can pay attention to how they lived and apply what makes sense. If you have the ability to align with nature, you absolutely fucking should. If not, do the best you can. Following nature's principles will get you pretty damn close.

In this chapter, I'm breaking down the sun's role in your biology and the key circadian hormones you should actually give a fuck about. And listen, I could go deep—*real* deep—on circadian hormones. There are layers to this and if you wanted to nerd out on every last detail, you could spend years studying it. But I'm not here to throw you into a hormonal dissertation. I'm here to make sure you *understand* how your body works so you can actually use this information.

There are a lot of circadian hormones, but I'm focusing on the big ones: insulin, cortisol, and melatonin. Why? Because they control your energy, metabolism, sleep, and overall ability to function like a human being instead of a half-dead zombie running on caffeine and sugar.

Before we dive into the hormones, however, let's give a brief overview of what circadian hormones even are in the first place.

CIRCADIAN HORMONES: YOUR BODY'S BUILT-IN CLOCK

Your body runs on rhythm—specifically, the circadian rhythm. This is your internal clock, a twenty-four-hour cycle that keeps everything in sync. It tells you when to wake up, when to eat, when to sleep, when to burn fat, when to store fat, and when to recover.

And the thing running the show? Light from the sun.

The sun doesn't just help you see—it literally programs your body. Every morning when the sun rises, it emits specific wavelengths of light that act as a biological alarm clock, telling your body it's time to start the day. Those light signals trigger the release of hormones like cortisol (your get-up-and-go hormone), melatonin (your rest-and-repair hormone), and insulin (your metabolic manager).

Now, even if you're inside, even if you're wearing clothes, even if your eyes are closed, your body still *senses* the sun's presence. Light penetrates your skin, your skull, even your bones. It's energy, frequency, and information all rolled into one.

And we used to be perfectly in sync with it. Our ancestors didn't need a biology degree to figure this out. They lived outside, walked barefoot, and let nature do its thing. They weren't staring at screens until midnight, wondering why they couldn't sleep. They weren't eating at random hours, throwing their entire system out of whack. They followed the light, and their bodies rewarded them for it.

Unfortunately, we've become completely disconnected. We live in artificial light, sleep in Wi-Fi-drenched rooms, and stare at blue-lit screens all day. We wear clothes made of plastic. We treat light like it's just a convenience when in reality, it's *life itself.*

And because we've removed ourselves from nature, our hormones are a mess. We're tired but wired, craving sugar all the time, unable to lose weight, and completely out of sync with our biological blueprint.

But let me remind you: You're not broken, girlfriend. You're just fighting against the natural rhythm your body is begging you to follow.

THE SUN IS PROGRAMMING YOU WHETHER YOU LIKE IT OR NOT

Think of your circadian rhythm like a GPS. Your body doesn't just *see* light—it *interprets* it. That's how it knows what time of day it is and what it should be doing. But if you're constantly bombarding yourself with artificial light at the wrong times and hiding from natural light when you actually need it, your GPS won't work right.

Here's what's happening at a biological level:

- Morning sunlight tells your body to wake up, burn fat, and regulate insulin properly.
- Midday sunlight helps you produce vitamin D and charges up your mitochondria.
- Evening light signals your body to start winding down for rest.
- But artificial light at night? That shit keeps your brain in daytime mode, wrecking your melatonin and keeping you in fat-storing survival mode.

Every hormone in your body is tied to these light signals. If you ignore them, you're setting yourself up for insulin resistance, shitty sleep, a wrecked metabolism, and brain fog so thick you'll swear you have early-onset dementia.

Now that you've got the basics on circadian hormones, let's dive into the three you need to obey: insulin, cortisol, and melatonin.

THE THREE CIRCADIAN HORMONES
INSULIN: THE GATEKEEPER OF FAT AND ENERGY

We covered a lot about insulin in Chapter 4, but now it's time to talk about this fat-storing hormone in the context of your circadian rhythm.

Most people treat insulin like an afterthought, something that only matters if you have diabetes or are counting calories. But that mindset is a huge fucking mistake. Insulin isn't just a passive player in your metabolism—it's the master regulator of what your body does with food.

Your body is naturally more insulin-sensitive in the morning, meaning it processes food more efficiently earlier in the day. This is because cortisol—your "get up and go" hormone—rises in the morning, signaling your body to release stored glucose for energy. Insulin works hand in hand with cortisol, ensuring that this energy gets where it needs to go.

But as the day progresses, insulin sensitivity declines. By evening, your body is shifting gears, winding down to prepare for repair and recovery. Insulin is supposed to step aside. But if you're eating late at night, you're forcing insulin to stick around longer than it should, and this throws everything off.

If insulin is still active when the sun goes down, it creates a hormonal traffic jam—and one of the biggest casualties is poor, little melatonin. Melatonin, your sleep hormone, can't fully do its job if insulin is still in the mix. Think of it like a bouncer at a club: you can't get in until insulin leaves (more on this in a second).

This is why eating late wrecks your sleep. If you've ever found yourself tossing and turning at night after a big dinner, this is why. Your body is still dealing with the metabolic consequences of food instead of shifting into repair mode. Worse, when melatonin production gets disrupted, you don't just get poor sleep, you disrupt everything from fat burning to immune function to hormone balance.

Giving your body the space to let insulin clear out means melatonin can show up on time, your body can focus on deep repair, and you wake up feeling like a sexy race car instead of a sluggish jalopy.

CORTISOL: NATURE'S ALARM CLOCK

Cortisol gets a bad rap, but it's not inherently a bad hormone. In fact, it's absolutely essential when your lifestyle aligns with nature. Cortisol is the hormone that gets your ass out of bed in the morning and puts you into action mode.

The trouble starts when you throw your body out of balance with constant stress, overconsumption of coffee, or a domesticated lifestyle that ignores natural rhythms. That's when cortisol can run wild, burning out your adrenal glands and leaving you in a mess.

As a part of your body's circadian rhythm, cortisol is most active during the day and naturally wanes at night. That's the ideal balance. You want cortisol to kick in and energize you in the morning, then calm down as evening approaches.

But for many women, that shit doesn't happen at all.

Let's start with cortisol's original job. It's your body's natural alarm system, releasing in the early morning to wake you up and prepare you for the day. Around 2:00 a.m., your cortisol releases slowly, gradually increasing as your body senses the first hints of light. By sunrise, cortisol is surging to help you wake up, and it even triggers glucagon, which releases glycogen stores from your liver to raise your blood sugar. This is often called the "dawn effect." That boost gives you the energy to start your day, but it's also why fasting in the morning doesn't make sense; your body is increasing your blood sugar naturally.

The dawn effect is nature's way of priming you for action. If we were still living in the wild, you'd wake up and immediately start moving—walking to a water source, gathering eggs, or preparing for the day's hunt. You'd eat your meals during the daylight hours because hunting in the dark wasn't an option. As the sun set, cortisol would fade, signaling your body to wind down and prepare for melatonin, your nighttime hormone, to take over.

Modern life, however, has flipped this natural rhythm on its head. Artificial light from phones and screens messes with cortisol's timing. Blue light from your screens mimics the sun's midday spectrum, tricking your brain into thinking it's still daytime. This keeps cortisol active and delays melatonin, disrupting your sleep and leaving you wired at the wrong times.

The dopamine hit from screens doesn't help either. Just like the blue sky makes you happy because of the dopamine released by natural light, synthetic blue light from your phone gives you a quick dopamine surge. But unlike nature's gentle rhythm, as you know from the last chapter, this hit is artificial and addictive, leading to dopamine toxicity. This can make you irritable and overstimulated.

When cortisol and dopamine are out of sync, it's a recipe for disaster. You're constantly chasing energy highs, burning out your body's natural systems, and breaking the delicate balance of your hormones.

This is why it's so critical to live in alignment with your body's natural programming.

Your body is designed to work with the sun's rhythms. That means waking up with cortisol, eating during the daylight hours, and letting melatonin (which we'll talk about next) take over as the sun sets. By sticking to this natural cycle, you support your hormones, keep cortisol in check, and set yourself up for better energy, sleep, and overall health.

MELATONIN: THE MITOCHONDRIA WHISPERER

People think of melatonin as just a sleep hormone, but it's so, so much more. Melatonin is one of the body's most powerful antioxidants. It cleans up damage, repairs tissue, and restores your cells.

Did you know you have two types of melatonin? You have day-time melatonin, which is made inside your cells (intracellular), and nighttime melatonin, which comes from your pineal gland.

But—and this is important—your body can only make that intra-cellular melatonin if you're exposed to sunlight.

Melatonin plays a vital role in keeping your mitochondria happy, and happy mitochondria are the key to a healthy, well-functioning body. Happy mitochondria don't just stop there either. They also communicate directly with your genes, programming how your cells function, and even how they repair themselves.

This is what you need to know: During the day, melatonin is pro-duced intracellularly within your mitochondria, acting as a protective agent. It soothes and repairs cellular damage, ensuring your cells stay healthy and your energy systems run smoothly. At night, melatonin shifts gears, being released extracellularly from the pineal gland to prepare your body for deep rest and cellular recovery. This dual action is critical for your overall health, because melatonin essentially man-ages your body's cleanup and restoration crew.

Like I mentioned earlier, melatonin and insulin don't get along. If you eat late at night, insulin comes out to process the food, and when insulin is present, melatonin can't do its job. It's like trying to run two competing programs on the same computer—it just doesn't work. Late-night eating sends insulin into overdrive, which blocks melatonin from being released and disrupts your body's ability to repair and recover while you sleep.

This is why timing matters so much. When you avoid eating at night, you allow melatonin to come out and get to work. Your mitochondria stay happy, your genes get their proper programming, and your body enters a restorative state that sets you up for peak performance the next day.

A NOTE ON SUPPLEMENTS

Here's another principle Tom and I try to follow: if your body is designed to make something, you shouldn't be taking it as a supplement.

But there are exceptions.

The real goal isn't to pop pills—it's to get your body producing what it needs naturally by fixing your environment and aligning with your circadian rhythms. Your body is a genius. It knows exactly what to do—if you stop fucking with nature.

Take melatonin, for example. Women are downing melatonin gummies like candy, desperate for sleep. But melatonin isn't just some over-the-counter sleep aid—it's a powerful circadian hormone your body produces on its own when it gets the right environmental cues. If you're constantly supplementing it, you're basically telling your body, "Don't bother making this anymore, I've got it covered."

That's not a long-term solution.

Instead of relying on melatonin supplements, fix the root problem. Ditch artificial light at night, stop eating late, and get outside during the day. Your body is fully capable of producing all the melatonin you need, if you let it. Relying on the gummy version is short-changing yourself.

Then there's vitamin D. This one's a bit different. The vast majority of people are vitamin D deficient, not because their bodies can't make it, but because they never go outside. We're cooped up indoors, disconnected from the sun—the very thing that triggers vitamin D production.

Vitamin D is one of the few supplements I give a pass to because 90 percent of people need it. But I want to be clear: sunlight is *always* better. It doesn't just give you vitamin D; it triggers a cascade of biological processes no supplement can replicate. So, while I won't shame you for taking vitamin D, remember, it's a crutch. The real solution is to get outside and soak up the sun.

It's the same story with other hormones your body is built to make, like testosterone. If you're mega-dosing synthetic vitamin D, downing melatonin, or relying on hormone replacements without addressing why your body isn't producing them naturally, you're missing the point.

Your body is like a perfectly designed program—all the pieces are there, if you let them work together. But if one piece isn't in the right place, the whole thing stalls. You can't patch that with supplements forever.

The real solution is to create an environment where your body can thrive. Get outside, let the sun program your system, and align yourself with nature's rhythms. When you give your body the right inputs—natural light, good sleep, real food—it knows exactly what to do (better than any pill ever could).

RECLAIMING YOUR RHYTHM

Modern life has turned us into Pottenger's cats—domesticated, fragile, and vitamin D deficient. We live under artificial light, slather ourselves in SPF 100, and only venture outside for a few minutes a day—fully clothed, of course. We've engineered a lifestyle that actively suppresses our ability to make the very hormones that keep us strong, healthy, and resilient. Then we wonder why we're anxious, inflamed, tired, and fat.

But your body still remembers. Beneath the cravings and brain fog and burnout is a primal rhythm just waiting to be restored.

You don't need a total life overhaul. You just need to start listening to the cues that have always been there: the sunrise, the urge to move, the natural pull toward rest. These are not random. They're your biological programming—and when you obey them, everything starts working the way it's supposed to.

This is what the principles are here for. To break the spell of domestication. To pull you out of the modern fog. To help you remember what it feels like to be alive in the way nature intended.

Because getting raw, sexy, and free isn't just a vibe.

It's what nature wants.

REIGNITE YOUR SEX LIFE

It's time to reignite your sex hormones, girlfriend! Because being a dried-up, cranky grandma ain't the vibe.

This chapter's going to be juicy. I love talking about sex drive because sex drives are a symbol that you're not going to age—not in the way the world expects, anyway. When your sex drive is lit up, it means your hormones are working, your energy is flowing, and your body is alive.

It's not just about wanting sex. It's about your vitality.

So what tanks your sex drive? Put simply: your hormones. And your hormones aren't just chemicals—they're your *personality*. They're your zest. They're your emotional range, your resilience, your desire. When your hormones crash, you don't just lose your libido, you lose the part of you that wants to dance, laugh, and flirt.

Your sex drive is the litmus test for how alive you are. It's not just about sex. It's your mood, your glow, and your hormones firing on all cylinders. When it's gone, you feel old and flat, like your vagina's been living in the desert.

No fucking thank you.

We're not meant to shrivel up and disappear after forty. But we've domesticated ourselves—made life too easy, too artificial, and paid the price with our hormones. That's why it's time to get wild again, baby!

This chapter is your invitation to stop settling for hormone chaos and start feeling alive in your sexy skin. We're going to tackle what's tanking your hormones and killing your sex drive, break down why menopause is *not* the end of your sex life, and give you real, doable steps to reignite your fire.

Buckle in, ladies!

WHAT KILLS YOUR HORMONES

Your sex hormones aren't just slacking off for no reason; they're responding to their environment. Modern life has created the perfect storm of stress, nutrient depletion through clown food, and disconnected relationships. And your poor hormones are doing their best to survive the chaos.

But survival mode is not sexy mode.

So if you're feeling blah, disinterested, or disconnected, it's not your fault—but it is your signal. Let's dig into the biggest culprits and get your inner fire roaring again.

LOW IODINE = HORMONAL MELTDOWN

Your sex glands can't function without iodine. That is a fact. Iodine is one of the key building blocks your body uses to make hormones. If you're deficient—and most women are—your thyroid tanks, your boobs get sore, your skin gets dry, and your vagina dries right up.

It's not just about dryness, though. Low iodine throws off your whole hormonal orchestra—thyroid, ovaries, breasts, adrenals. They all suffer. And when your thyroid isn't humming, your metabolism stalls, your mood flatlines, and yes, your sex drive crashes.

Most women have never been told this. That's why I recommend the book *The Iodine Crisis* by Lynne Farrow. It will blow your mind. She breaks down how iodine deficiency is linked to breast cancer, fibroids, cysts, and hormone chaos. She also shares how to safely replenish your iodine levels.

Seaweed, seafood, and quality iodine supplements (like Lugol's) are your new BFFs—just be sure to talk to your doctor before starting iodine. My favorite doctor and resource on the subject is Dr. David Brownstein.

LOW VITAMIN D = LOW EVERYTHING

Vitamin D isn't just for bones; it's an important hormone that regulates your big three: estrogen, progesterone, and testosterone. When women come to me complaining about mood swings, hot flashes, low progesterone, and zero sex drive, one of the first things I ask is, "What are your vitamin D levels?"

Nine times out of ten, they say, "It's in the thirties."

Girl. That's not a green light. That's a hormonal slow death.

Your vitamin D levels should be at sixty or higher if you want your body to thrive, not just scrape by. Because—and this is important—vitamin D is like the ignition switch for your hormonal engine. Without it, your body can't convert cholesterol into sex hormones. You can be eating clean, taking all the right supplements, doing everything "right," but if your D is low, your spark won't catch.

Vitamin D also helps regulate your immune system, your mood, your sleep, your skin, and your inflammation levels. It is sunshine in hormone form. When your vitamin D level is low, that means your cellular energy is low, which means no sex drive.

How do you fix this? Follow Principle #5, of course: worship the sun! That's right—this isn't just about taking a supplement and calling it a day. Your body *needs* real light, real warmth, and real UVB rays. Get outside. Let the sunlight hit your skin and your eyes first thing in the morning. This tells your brain to wake up, boosts your serotonin, and helps regulate your entire hormonal rhythm.

If sunlight isn't always an option, then yes, use a quality D3 supplement or even a vitamin D lamp in the darker months. But don't forget, supplements are just stand-ins for the real thing. Getting your D levels up is one of the fastest ways to feel sexy, sane, and switched back on.

EXCESSIVE CORTISOL = BYE-BYE SEX DRIVE

While addressing low iodine and low vitamin D is relatively easy to do, addressing stress levels is a whole other ballgame. And we all know that high stress means high cortisol.

High cortisol is the ultimate hormone killer. It's your body's emergency broadcast system, and when it's always on, your hormones go offline because your body prioritizes survival over pleasure. If it thinks you're running from a tiger (or just juggling a job, kids, a to-do list from hell, and no sleep), it's not going to waste energy on making you feel sexy.

And cortisol overload isn't just from emotional stress. It's from *overstimulating yourself all day long.* Blue light at night. Scrolling TikTok or Instagram in bed. Not eating meat, pounding coffee, and pretending like sleep is optional. Every one of those things spikes cortisol and drains your progesterone.

Coffee especially is a sneaky little sex drive saboteur. I know, I know—it feels like a hug in a mug. But let's call it what it is: coffee is a drug. And like any drug, it comes with a cost. Coffee isn't just a casual pick-me-up; it's a whip to a tired horse. And guess who the horse is? You. Every time you sip that mug, you're forcing your already-exhausted body to perform. You're not giving yourself more energy; you're borrowing against tomorrow. And what's the cost? Your sex hormones. Coffee spikes cortisol, and chronic cortisol is a known hormone killer. It tells your body to prioritize survival over reproduction, leaving your libido, your glow, and your hormonal balance in the dust.

You can keep your cup, but understand the trade-off—it will

rob you of your sex hormones. Excessive caffeine keeps your cortisol chronically high. You may feel alert, but on the inside, your hormones are withering.

This is why many women hit forty and suddenly can't sleep, can't focus, and can't get turned on. Their adrenals are cooked, their sex hormones have left the building, and coffee is a big part of that burnout.

And it doesn't stop there. Coffee is highly acidic, it dehydrates you, and it accelerates aging. That glow you're chasing gets dulled by coffee. The smooth, youthful skin you work so hard to protect breaks down faster under its dehydrating, acid-forming effects.

I've worked with thousands of women and when they quit coffee, their hormones improve across the board. I believe lived experience speaks louder than studies.

But you get to choose: the temporary buzz or your long-term beauty and vitality. I know which one matters to me more.

MICROBES = SILENT MOOD (AND LIBIDO) KILLERS

Let's talk about your gut—and your man's gut, for that matter. Your microbiome isn't just about digestion; it's one of the main regulators of your immune system, your mood, your inflammation levels, and yes, your hormones. Your gut bugs are running the show behind the scenes and if they're out of balance, you're going to feel off, anxious, bloated, and definitely not in the mood.

Now here's where it gets interesting: your microbes are picky about who they mate with. If your husband's got a gut full of beer, Doritos, and drive-through microbes, your body *knows*. Your good microbes don't want to mix with his bad microbes. So what happens? You pull away. You stop wanting to have sex with him. Not because you're not attracted to him, but because your microbes are literally repelled.

I've seen this happen over and over in my own life. Back when my gut was a mess, I attracted men whose guts were a mess too.

I have two ex-husbands who were beer-drinking, fast food-eating, microbially-disastrous partners. At the time, I didn't know it, but I had bad microbes too, so of course I was attracted to them. I didn't realize it then, but my body was saying, "Yep, we're the same kind of toxic mess."

As I healed in subsequent years, my body literally started rejecting people's energy, their smell, and even their touch. It sounds woo-woo, but it's straight biology. The healthier I got, the more I couldn't stand the smell, energy, or presence of certain people because our microbes were no longer a match.

But here's the good news: you can change that. Start feeding both of your guts the good stuff. You already know that fermented foods are important—we learned that back in Chapter 2. Start eating all the ferments—sauerkraut, kimchi, kefir, pickled onions, raw cheeses. Most guys enjoy these foods. If not, serve them with a steak or with some eggs. The healthier his microbes get, the more your body will say, "Yes, please."

And this still matters even if you're single, ladies. A happy gut makes for a happy libido. If your microbiome is thriving, your mood will lift, your brain will work better, and your hormones will sing. That's hot. That's attractive. That's how you show up sexy AF without even trying.

And this whole microbe thing? It's not just about who you sleep with. It's about who you spend your time around too. Your microbial environment is constantly being shaped by the people you share space with. Nurses and hospital workers often pick up the microbes of the unhealthy patients they care for. People who work in gyms swap microbes with everyone sweating on equipment. Even hanging out at a friend's house where someone eats junk and lives in a stressed-out body can shift your terrain.

Research is starting to show what ancient cultures already knew: community is biological. Your body responds to your environment on a microscopic level. So be mindful of who you breathe around, who you hug, and who you let in your home. Your microbes are listening.

LACK OF GOOD SEX = LACK OF HORMONE STIMULATION

If you're not enjoying sex, your hormones are going to peace out. That whole "use it or lose it" thing is real. Your body is constantly listening and taking notes. If you're going through the motions without pleasure, it assumes sex isn't a priority and starts shutting that whole system down.

So let's call it out: bad sex is bad for your health. And martyr sex—where you're doing it just to check a box or keep the peace—is worse. Your body is smart. If you're giving but not receiving, your hormones aren't going to bother showing up. They need a reason. They need the spark. And that comes from you getting turned on and feeling *sexy*.

Now, what if your husband isn't showing up for you? What if he's checking out after his climax, doing the same old routine, or not even asking what you want? Well, it's time for a grown-up conversation, girlfriend. We are not little girls here. We are grown-ass women. And grown-ass women don't fake orgasms. Instead, they instruct. They say, "Lower. Slower. Do that again." They grab a hand. They move his mouth. They take the lead.

If that sounds out of your comfort zone, just know that most men *want* to please their wives. They just need some guidance. So stop being a martyr. Stop being quiet. Stop hoping he'll magically figure it out. Instead, talk dirty to him! Seriously. Your husband is going to love it. He's been dying for you to be more vocal, more playful, and more bold. Don't be afraid to let that wild, sexy part of you take the mic.

LACK OF ORGASM = NO INCENTIVE

I've said this a lot, but it bears repeating: Your body is smart. It truly is brilliant. It knows when you're not getting the reward, and it responds by shutting down the system that's supposed to generate the desire. Without an orgasm, there's no incentive. Why would your body keep pouring energy into a hormonal cocktail meant to get you in the mood if there's no big finish?

When you don't orgasm, your body interprets sex as a waste of energy. It's just another chore, another box to check. And guess what? Your hormones start dialing it in too. Progesterone? Meh. Testosterone? Nah. Estrogen? Maybe next cycle. Your libido doesn't just vanish; it gets buried under resentment, fatigue, and a sea of unmet needs.

Orgasms matter (maybe we should put *that* on a shirt!). Not because it's about performance or pressure, but because your pleasure is a signal. It tells your body, "Yes, this is good. Let's do more of this." It boosts oxytocin, lowers cortisol, and helps you make more sex hormones.

It's the same concept when we discussed insulin: If you never eat carbs, your body stops producing insulin because it doesn't need to. If you never orgasm, your body assumes sex isn't important and stops producing sex hormones too. Your biology runs on demand. No stimulation? No production. So yes, your orgasm is part of your hormonal strategy. If you don't use it, you lose it—literally.

You have to connect to *your* pleasure again. Explore. Get curious. Use your hands. Use a toy. Let go of shame. And for the love of all things juicy, communicate. If he's not helping you get there, you have to speak up. Guide him. Show him. You are not a passive passenger in your sex life. Be the driver.

And just so I'm clear: you're never too old to French kiss. I don't care if you've been together thirty years or you've got grandkids. Your husband's saliva contains testosterone, and when that mixes with your biology, it turns you *on*. That's not just sexy, it's science.

So kiss, play, and touch his naughty bits.

THE MENOPAUSE MYTH

There's a cultural lie that after menopause, women are supposed to shut down. No more sex. No more intimacy. Just shrivel up and start wearing beige.

How about a big fat no!

Somewhere along the way, we decided that menopause was the

end of the road. That if you're not ovulating anymore, then clearly you have no business being sexy, desirable, or fully embodied. But let me tell you something: menopause is not your expiration date. Instead, let it be your queen era!

At menopause and beyond, you are royalty. You're wiser. Freer. You know who you are. You're not living for approval anymore. You don't care about being polite all the time. And you sure as hell don't have to accept that your sex life is over.

If you've lost the desire, the drive, or the connection, that doesn't mean it's gone forever. It just means something needs your attention. Is it hormones? Is it resentment? Is it boredom? Is it body shame? Is it a partner who doesn't show up anymore?

These are the years when you're meant to be in full bloom. You're the matriarch now. The fire doesn't die; it just moves deeper into your bones. So stop accepting dryness as your destiny. Stop believing the lie that you've aged out of pleasure. You were made for pleasure, for connection, and for feeling good.

This is where you get to reinvent it all. Let your next chapter be your hottest one yet.

BECOMING THE MATRIARCH

Did you know that humans are one of only a handful of species that go through menopause? And that we are the only ones who live decades beyond it?

Killer whales and elephants are two of the few species where older females take on leadership roles after their reproductive years—through either menopause or lifelong matriarchy. In killer whale pods, when the oldest females stop reproducing, they become the *leaders* of the group. They guide migration patterns. They teach the young. They help the pod survive. In times of crisis—drought, starvation, disorientation—it's the postmenopausal females who save the group.

It's the same with elephants. The matriarch leads the herd. She's the memory keeper, the decision maker, the protector. She's not the weakest link; she's the one everyone turns to when shit hits the fan. And she doesn't do it with a clipboard and a frown. She does it with power, presence, and instinct.

That's you. Or at least—it *could* be you, if you follow this principle.

You can't step into your matriarch energy if you're exhausted, disconnected, and dried up. You've got to be turned on—not just sexually, but spiritually, mentally, and emotionally. People don't follow a woman who is burned out and bitter. They follow the woman who is lit from within. Who laughs deeply. Who speaks with authority and compassion. Who knows how to flirt *and* fight for her family.

Becoming the matriarch isn't about becoming quiet and soft and saintly. It's about becoming *unignorable*. Not because you're shouting, but because your sex hormones haven't been ignored. You are fully in your power. That is sexy. That is rare. And that is what makes people—partners, kids, grandkids, communities—pay attention.

So if you want to be the woman everyone turns to, the woman everyone respects, the woman your partner still drools over after forty or fifty years, you have to wake up your inner matriarch. You have to feel good in your body. You have to honor the wisdom in your blood. And you have to stop buying the lie that it's too late.

Because it's not.

HOW TO REIGNITE YOUR FIRE

Now that we've called out all the things that tank your hormones, let's talk about what brings them back to life. This isn't about perfection; it's about momentum. Tiny shifts with big ripple effects. You don't need to overhaul your life in one night, but you *do* need to start choosing actions that send the signal: "Hey body, it's safe to feel good again."

What follows is your tool kit. These are the practices, foods, and mindset shifts that tell your system it's time to wake up, warm up, and get turned on. Pick one and commit. Then add another. Stack the habits, stack the wins.

I covered the basics earlier, but here's a quick reminder:

- Get your vitamin D above sixty.
- Do your research on iodine and see if it's right for you.
- Watch your stress levels.
- Ditch the coffee addiction.
- Build a healthy gut (for you and your partner) by eating fermented foods.

Now let's get into the juicy stuff. Because healing your hormones isn't just about lab tests and supplements, it's about reconnecting with the part of you that *feels alive*. This section is all about turning the lights back on in your relationship, your body, and your energy field. And I'm not talking about lingerie and candles (though those can be fun too). I'm talking about real, playful, and primal intimacy that wakes up your nervous system and makes your hormones say, "Oh hell yes, we're back."

These aren't just cute date night tips. These are hormone-rebooting, spark-reviving practices that remind your body what it's like to be turned on by life, love, and touch.

- **Hug and kiss your partner.** For real, though. I'm not talking about a drive-by smooch. I'm talking a real embrace—the kind that says, "I still choose you." Hold it longer than you think you should. Let your bodies sync. This releases oxytocin, lowers cortisol, and starts to bring the emotional safety that makes desire possible.
- **Touch more. Flirt. Be playful.** If you haven't slapped his butt in a while, it's time. Play footsie. Steal kisses. Slow dance. Text something flirty in the middle of the day. Think back to your teenage years when dry humping was fun and a total turn on. Be playful and fun. Get creative.
- **French kiss!** Don't overthink it. Just grab him and go. It doesn't have to lead anywhere (although it probably will, let's be real),

but that deep kiss sends a signal to your nervous system that connection is happening. Plus, as I mentioned before, his saliva contains testosterone, which literally turns you on. You're never too old to make out like teenagers!

- **Let him smell you.** Your natural scent is part of the attraction equation. Skip the overperfumed stuff and let your real pheromones do their job. If you like his scent, great. If you don't, it might be his gut talking. A few weeks of fermented foods can do wonders.
- **Get dirty and stay dirty.** Seriously. Skip the shower post-sex or after a workout and just *exist* with each other's scents. Let your primal chemistry do its work. This is how you reconnect on a raw, instinctual level. And when you do shower, shower together and rub up on one another.

Meow!

YOUR ANCESTORS WERE SEXY, YOU SHOULD BE TOO

What you just read in this chapter isn't just about sex; it's about *vitality*. It's about reclaiming something ancient, something primal, something you were born with.

Your ancestors were sexy. They danced under the moon. They gave birth in huts, not sterile hospitals. They moved their bodies with rhythm. They flirted, they laughed, they played, and they didn't question whether they were "too old" to feel alive. They *knew* that sexuality was part of health, not separate from it.

You come from that lineage.

And I get it—modern life has tried to domesticate that part of you. Hormones tank, libido disappears, and next thing you know, you're wondering if sweatpants and resentment are just the next phase of adulthood.

I refuse to believe that shit, though. You should refuse too.

It's time to reclaim your spark. Flirt again. Kiss again. Say yes to life again. Because getting sexy isn't about six-pack abs or perfect hair. It's about being *fully alive* in your body, your energy, and your pleasure.

So get sexy, girlfriend! Your hormones are ready for their comeback.

CONCLUSION

You were meant to feel sexy.

Not just in your twenties, but throughout your entire life. Not just occasionally with the lights off. You were built to feel alive in your skin—turned on, magnetic, radiant. That's your natural state.

But we've strayed so far from nature that it's hard to believe that feeling sexy is even possible anymore. We've been trained to expect a slow decline. To normalize the fatigue, the weight gain, the low libido, the brain fog. To laugh it off with, "Well, I guess this is just what getting older feels like."

That is all bullshit.

You were never meant to deteriorate. You were never meant to dim. You were designed to evolve into a stronger, wiser, more vibrant version of yourself. That includes feeling sexy. Because sexiness is vitality, and vitality is health.

We've been taught to settle. To call it "normal" when we can't sleep, can't focus, can't fit into our jeans. We've been programmed to accept aging as inevitable problems and shittiness. That our bodies are the enemy and our biology is something to fight.

That is all still bullshit.

Your body has always been on your side. It's been trying to communicate with you all along. The bloating, the brain fog, the low libido, the stubborn weight—these are not flaws; they're feedback.

And now you know how to listen.

This book—*Get Sexy, Girlfriend! Your Ancestors Were Attractive and You Should Be Too*—was never about discipline or willpower. It was a reminder that *you are nature.* You are not separate from it—you *are* it. You were built to burn fat, to sleep deeply, to feel joy, to heal, to move with energy and intention. Your body was designed to vibrate with life. You weren't meant to shuffle through your days feeling numb, puffy, anxious, and exhausted. You were meant to prance, to glow, to feel so good that you can't help but say, "Holy shit, this is what health feels like."

This book wasn't about hacks or fads. It was a return to the truth your body has known all along. The 7 Principles of Nature weren't invented in a lab or dreamed up on a whiteboard. They're written in your cells.

So what did we learn? Let's recap.

- **Principle #1: Don't Fuck with Nature.** She always wins. Align with her or suffer the consequences.
- **Principle #2: Don't Eat Clown Food.** You're not a science experiment. Eat like a human, not a lab rat.
- **Principle #3: Find Joy Outside of Food.** Food isn't your therapist. Find joy through experiences with loved ones that you can take to the grave.
- **Principle #4: Master Your Fuel Systems—or Stay Fat and Tired.** Your body is a fat-burning beast. Stop clogging the engine with sugar.
- **Principle #5: Worship the Sun.** You're solar-powered. The sun is your charger, not your enemy.
- **Principle #6: Obey Your Circadian Clock.** Your body runs on light and darkness. Disrespect it and everything becomes harder.
- **Principle #7: Reignite Your Sex Life.** Aging doesn't kill desire,

neglect does. Bring back the spark and become the matriarch you were meant to be.

Following the principles of nature isn't about perfection. But once you start living by them, you'll notice the difference, the big changes. Your body will wake up, your skin will glow, and your hormones will start singing again. You'll drop the bloat, the brain fog, and the bullshit. You'll stop managing symptoms and start radiating vitality.

You'll get sexy, like your ancestors.

You've been conditioned to believe that feeling like shit is normal by a system that profits from your pain. That story ends here. And no, you are never too old. Whether you're twenty, forty, or seventy-five, it's never too late.

In fact, the most perfect time is now.

Most people don't even know what "good" feels like. They're stuck in "okay," comparing themselves to other exhausted, inflamed humans. But okay is not good enough. You were made for *holy-shit-this-is-amazing* levels of health.

And when you get there—and you will—you'll stop treating your body like something to fix and start treating it like something to honor. Your body is a fancy race car, girlfriend. It's time to treat it as such.

So what now?

Start with the 7 Principles of Nature. Start small, but start *now*. Pick the one that speaks to you most and apply it today. Then build from there. Let momentum build. Progress is powerful.

Join the movement. If you want deeper support, we've got you. Head to PrimalBod.com for personalized coaching, expert guidance, and a badass community of women who refuse to settle.

Stay connected. Find us on Instagram, YouTube, or wherever you scroll. We're not going anywhere.

Share this book with a friend or loved one.

And most importantly—**lead your family**. Change what happens under your roof. Show your kids what real health looks like. Let them see you glowing. Let them see you prancing. Let them feel what it's like to be raised by someone who's living fully in their bodies. Because if you don't teach them, someone else will. And that someone could be the school lunch program, the food industry, or a pediatrician with a prescription pad. You've done the unlearning so they don't have to.

You've spent enough time disconnected from the earth beneath your feet, the sun in the sky, and the rhythms that once guided your every cell. But now you know the truth—and once you know, you can't un-know.

So, follow the principles. Let them lead you back to yourself—back to the way you were meant to live before modern life pulled you off track: wild, primal, and sexy as hell.

ACKNOWLEDGMENTS

Thanks to our Chief Storytelling Girlfriend, Aleks Mendel, for helping me write this book.

To our incredible Primal Bod members—the rest of the Girlfriends—thank you for taking a chance on me.

And to our amazing team: thank you for helping Tom and I deliver on the most successful weight-loss program out there. We couldn't do it without you!

ABOUT THE AUTHORS

CANDI FRAZIER

Candi Frazier is board-certified in holistic nutrition, a natural weight-loss expert, and co-founder of Primal Bod—the most successful weight-loss program ever created, empowering individuals to achieve sustainable health through education. With more than a decade of experience in functional nutrition and holistic wellness, Candi specializes in helping women reclaim their physique by aligning their habits with nature-based principles. Her personal journey of overcoming health struggles inspired her to create Primal Bod alongside her husband, Tom—a program that has transformed thousands of lives. Candi's no-nonsense approach to nutrition, paired with her deep connection to clients, has made her a trusted leader in the weight-loss industry. Known for helping women get bikini-ready—physically and emotionally—Candi's mission is to guide women toward vibrant, primal living.

THOMAS FRAZIER

Thomas Frazier is an entrepreneur and co-founder of Primal Bod. With a background in finance and business strategy, Tom pairs his reverence for nature with his knowledge of insulin as a type 1 diabetic to clarify the Primal Bod message. His work with Candi blends sharp business acumen with a deep passion for helping people shift their paradigms about epigenetics and the truth of how the body works. Before co-founding Primal Bod, Tom built a career as a CPA, where his financial expertise helped him navigate and grow various ventures.

Outside of work, Candi and Tom enjoy spending time in the great outdoors with their blended family. They live in Wisconsin and have five children between them. Learn more about Candi, Tom, and Primal Bod at PrimalBod.com.